The Real Life Story of Stem Cells

About the Authors

Dr. Bhaskar Vyas (1937) Plastic Surgeon and Dr. Rajni Vyas (1937) Obstetrician and Gynecologist have contributed to their respective fields with research innovations. Dr. R. Vyas has made a seminal contribution to unexplained reproductive failure with a success rate of 55% with her research protocol. This is highest success rate. Dr. B. Vyas' seminal contribution is to derive several products from stem cells obtained from fat. They have numerous research papers published. They have published over a score of books. Concept Publishing Company has published their books on the topic of philosophy, psychology and physics viz. 'Contemporizing Raj Yoga', 'Experiments with Truth and Non-violence – China Challenged' 3rd Edition, 'Indian Handbook of Hypnotherapy' 4th Edition, Space Time Consciousness – Rationale of the Paranormal'. They are now working on a philosophical concept, 'Pragnya', to take it to an utilitarian application as 'Pragnya Quotient'. They finally introduced themselves as perennial students of philosophy.

The Real Life Story of Stem Cells

Dr. Bhaskar Vyas
and
Dr. Rajni Vyas

CONCEPT PUBLISHING COMPANY PVT. LTD.
NEW DELHI-110059

ISBN-13: 978-93-5439-066-1 (HB)

ISBN-13: 978-93-5439-067-8 (PB)

First Published 2021

Published and Printed by

Concept Publishing Company Pvt. Ltd.
A/15-16, Commercial Block, Mohan Garden,
New Delhi-110059 (India)
T: 91 11 41101460, 91 11 25351460, 91 11 25351794
E : publishing@conceptpub.com, *W*: www.conceptpub.com

Cataloging in Publication Data--Courtesy: D.K. Agencies (P) Ltd. <docinfo@dkagencies.com>

Vyas, Bhaskar, author.
The real life story of stem cells / Dr. Bhaskar Vyas and Dr. Rajni Vyas.
pages cm
Includes index.
ISBN 9789354390661 (HB)
ISBN 9789354390678 (PB)

1. Stem cells--Research--India. 2. Vyas, Bhaskar. 3. Vyas, Rajni. I. Vyas, Rajni, author. II. Title.

LCC QH588.S83V93 2021 | DDC 616.027740954 23

Foreword

Stem cell therapy has a long gestation period since the first stem cell was identified in the early twentieth century. It is almost a hundred years that the discovery process passed through different stages of identification, description of properties, isolation of stem cells, and finally, the application of stem cell therapy for therapeutic purpose or regenerative medicine in the twenty-first century. One could explain this delay in terms of several factors. It is not only due to the promulgation of germ theory and antibiotic revolution that pushed the biological diseases to the background for a long period but also because of the impact of the World War-II and changing state and science relationship. After the demonstration of power that the detonation of nuclear weapons generated and expressed in terms of the fetishism of force that the physical sciences gained greater public visibility and consequently greater funding at the neglect of biological sciences. This was also reflected in the reward system and the discovery of every new particle was honoured with a Nobel prize in the subsequent decades even if it became a routine science. A positive outcome was that the World War-II gave rise to ethical concerns for medical research and led to the establishment of the Nuremberg Code for human experimentation to combat racism or Nazi ideology. Finally, this movement evolved into the Helsinki Declaration and several revisions till 2013. However, Science got divorced from values or ethics and scientists started eschewing social responsibility for the application of science that they evolved.

It was not until the eighties that the biological sciences restored some respectability and that ushered into the biotechnology revolution. Along with this, the other technologies that emerged were information and communication technologies and nanotechnologies. These technologies co-evolved with an intertwined phenomenon of globalisation and the international environmental movement. Biotechnologies revolutionised the health sector and promised to treat several intractable diseases. At the same time, this phenomenon posed several challenges of social, economic, political, legal, and ethical nature. During this period ethics also re-entered the realm of science.

Curiosity in stem cell research was further kindled with the disentanglement of properties such as self-renewal and potency. Unlike plant stem cells that could be differentiated into any cell, the animal stem cells have different potency like totipotent, pluripotent, multipotent, and that only totipotent stem cells could be differentiated into any organism. More importantly, the totipotent stem cells were found only in embryos. After 1999, scientists discovered that manipulating adult mouse tissues could produce different cell types, and later the first embryonic stem cell lines of a human cell were derived. It was the use of human embryos that mainly raised ethical concerns. The understanding of cell biology also improved that led to the reprogramming of adult stem cells into totipotent stem cells reducing the ethical burden. It is after this period that stem cell research picked up momentum and there was a proliferation of stem cell research and clinics for stem cell therapy the world over. This included not only a genuine quest for research and therapies but also the world witnessed a proliferation of rogue clinics exploiting gullible patients including donors/vendors of oocytes of from women belonging to vulnerable sections. Many of these clinics advertised and promised unproven treatment. Different countries have followed different kinds of regulatory regimes ranging from restrictive to liberal regime leaving space for many researchers or doctors for their overzealous pursuits. The technological spread of stem cell therapies did not remain confined to the metropolitan centres of the advanced countries but there was rapid diffusion in the developing countries including India. This was reflected in an increasing number of research publications and patenting activity.

India figures as amongst the top fifteen countries as far as world publication ranking is concerned.

Given the wider socio-economic implications of these technologies, a need for socio-economic studies became imperative as well. I also started studying this phenomenon from a science policy and innovation system perspective along with my Ph.D. students. I had also undertaken a collaborative research project with a prestigious university in the UK. It was during this time almost a decade back while I was visiting my hometown Vadodara that I came across a newspaper report about a doctor who was engaged in stem cell research and therapy. My curiosity was fuelled by astonishment that doctors were dealing with an emerging area of science and technology in a relatively 'small town' called Vadodara. The upshot is that that in the globalized world the technological diffusion is rapid and the technological gap between the advanced countries and developing world was not wide in the emerging technologies. I could not resist calling him up for an appointment. This was Dr. Bhaskar Vyas, a plastic surgeon of international repute, who immediately granted me the interview, and the very next day allowed me to visit his clinic-*cum*-lab and discuss the implications of stem cell research. This professional association continued later with several seminars and meetings where he agreed to participate.

Recently, to my great delight, he approached me to write a foreword to his memoirs surrounding his work on stem cell research. As far as autobiographies and memoirs are concerned, it is easy to find many scientists publishing autobiographies but it is not so common to find such work authored by doctors or medical researchers. Here, you have memoirs penned by him and his wife Dr. Rajni and a short chapter contributed by their daughter from the UK. This work describes their journey through an uphill task of stem cell research and challenges that are faced by any pioneers. They have a racy style of writing that is iterative at times and jumps that make the readers think and captivate their imagination. It is about the unknown and unravelling of stem cell science. The book begins with their jousting over bureaucratic controls and overcoming the hurdles and about people who understood the value of stem cell research and extended a helping hand. The path of narration meanders at times into experiences of meeting great doctors and researchers or at time bursts into poetic expression and philosophical twists or into finer details of stem cell science that would interest specialists as well as any common reader.

These memoirs compel readers to rethink or redefine the ethical guidelines for stem cell research aimed at balancing between the urgency of medical need and abuse of this new science and technology and commodification of human organs. The socio-economic, ethical issues and risks are further compounded by the allied and emerging technologies such as gene editing. This technology involves greater risk while editing heritable characteristics. The complexities involved will certainly rummage the minds of inquisitive scholars. Finally, I leave the readers to ride the horses of dreams along with the authors.

August 8, 2020

Pranav N. Desai
Former Professor,
Centre for Studies in Science Policy
School of Social Sciences,
Jawaharlal Nehru University,
New Delhi

Contents

1
Genesis of the Beginning: The Source of Inspiration—"WHO?"

This autobiography is about the work of two comrades. Comrades in arms. When we decided to be life partners, it happened at an academic conference. Yes, there would have been romance, love, family relationships, bonding and convergence of consciousness to the extent of consilience. There were discussions, debates, dialectical discursions and difference in opinions but when it came to act, there was total agreement and unity. But the most precious ingredient of this conjugal relationship is comradeship. Comradeship in action. Neither of us alone would have been able to accomplish any one of the real life stories recited herein.

It should be remembered that the autobiography is about the life and work of two persons: What is accomplished has been conceptualized mainly by me and effortless eloquent execution has been done by Rajni. One would not be complete without the other. Before narrating further, we need to make one clarification. Autobiography by its very nature is written in a first person singular. However, there is radical departure here. This is the real life story of two persons. This has been happening all throughout our lives since we began to live together. For simplification the narration would be by me. But it implies a masterly execution by Rajni. Moreover, let us not enter into dialectical discussion as to whether happenings occur like a descent from the sky or they can be manipulated as a structure. It is certain that this story happens to be written by the application of multiple, multifaceted intelligences. A countless number of high profile scientists and several young brilliant scientists contributed to the development of the full story. The story has impacted their lives.

Stem cell research is like an ocean. Ocean has no beginning and no end. Its depth is variable. There are numerous pebbles on the seashore. This real life story concerns about our gathering a few pebbles as we walk on the beach and wet our feet with sea water.

Regardless, what Krishnamurty said about a pathless land, it is true over here also: the first step is the last step. Therefore, each chapter is readable as an independent short story and so all chapters are numbered as 1.

Before 5000 years, some 'Rishis' heard voices from the sky. Whatever may be their state of consciousness, they remembered what they heard. It was passed on verbally from generations to generations since there was no script. The first of the Vedas, 'Rig-Veda' is described as "voice heard from the sky" from divine origin—'*Apaurusha—not authored by any human being*'.

The 'Rishis' conceived that individual minds may also get interconnected. A state of high connectivity between human beings would then give rise to a cosmic web. It was conceptualized to exist universally and the mind was thought to be a receiver like radio. Therefore, 'Rishis' prayed, "Let noble thoughts come to us from all the sides." Significant as it is, 'Rig-Veda' does not describe any God or Goddess but what is stated is undoubtedly eternal truth. This may be so when understood in a poetic sense. Most people would like to call it instinct. This is a fundamental attribute of all human beings. When subscribed to by giant individuals like Mahatma Gandhi it may be called as a voice within. A modern age 'Rishi' may poetically illustrate it as, 'a moment reveals what heavens toiled to express for ages.' The aim of the present work is not to engage in this kind of dialectical, philosophical discussion. The work is about a simple answer that we have sought as a quest. Yet, not to find and yet not to yield; and search endlessly without accepting defeat. Thus, it is a story about our pursuit for the answer to derive from our stumbling into the field of stem cell research.

We Indians somehow or other have this trait of sky gazing and hearing voices from "Above". This has happened to us and that is how we sat down to write this story. There were several different paradigms that could become a good love story full of romance, passion and disappointment, there were times full of adventure, fulfilment of ambitions and failures and there were times when dreams did come true or significantly crash. We have never thought any one of them to be of important to write. There is nothing to eulogize but most situations have had a human face to show. Human faces that were full of aspirations, hopes, surety to endeavour and ability to withstand bad weather as well as gratuitous graces and munificent magnanimities that showed up spontaneously. We thought such a portrait gallery may be with indistinct faces of the authors, but full of vigour with the participants engaged. That would make a good gallery to show.

We have been believers in some kind of "divine design". When the events materialize from nowhere and catapult into a structural design, we would call them a happening. Scenic amongst my friends and readers would frown, "happenings? What divine design?"

But the aim of writing this is simply to tell a story. There is no aim to prove any scientific point of view whether the story is science or philosophy or both. As Carl Jung has written these are just happening.

Our basic training is in the discipline of science. We wondered at the physicality of matter and speculated about how the basic chemical elements got as rhythmically arranged as described by **Mendeleev**. When we trained as medical students, we were amazed how a malarial parasite will find its way into red blood corpuscles, multiply and in turn can be killed by a small pill.

Study in a medical school was for us an experience like Alice had in 'Wonderland'. Every bit of knowledge that we gathered was inculcated in our minds with a sense of wonder, surprise, astonishment and awe. A transformation occurs in the consciousness with these kinds of mental vibrations.

Sri Aurobindo has beautifully described this wonderland as follows:

In the blue of the sky, in the green of the forest,
Whose is the hand that has painted the glow?

When the winds were asleep in the womb of the ether,
Who was it roused them and bade them to blow?

He is lost in the heart, in the cavern of Nature,
He is found in the brain where He builds up the thought:
In the pattern and bloom of the flowers He is woven,
In the luminous net of the stars He is caught.

Sri Aurobindo, titled the poem as 'Who'. In his poetic effulgence, he carries his search with 5 more stanzas and finds him sitting alone in the darkness thus:

When darkness was blind and engulfed within darkness,
He was seated within it immense and alone.

Yet, we derived the inspiration with further question, such as what, how, and when that man sitting in the darkness alone seems to be working all the time. This is the factual genesis of this real life story of stem cells.

We cited the poem since we found Sri Aurobindo advocating on our behalf that whether happenings happen or divine design exists or not, it can certainly be seen as a shadow in a bright moonlight.

However, philosophy is the mother of all disciplines. A myth or a fantasy may also transform into philosophy when chiselled with sharp logic. Fantasy so occurs that, at times someone may fool around most people, most of the times. Charles Darwin (1809-1882) travelled across the globe on the ship, 'Beagle' collecting the fossils from several islands to come out with a brilliant hypothesis—"Theory of Evolution".

At this point Vatsal stopped transcripting and looking intently at me, he asked:

"So, the theory of evolution is a hoax?"

"No, there is no hoax. Evolution is a philosophical concept that has no empirical evidence."

"The fossils collected by Darwin are not evidence?"

"There is no empirical evidence that your parents were monkeys and tracing the ancestry to the limits of your family memory, there would not be any. Science today accepts evidence even for sub-atomic particles. To produce that kind of evidence, Charles Darwin will need to reincarnate again and again and produce a videographic film of transition. Therefore, let us not waste time in brilliant philosophical hypothecation."

Suffice it is to say that the logistic triggered a few geniuses.

With such a brilliant exposition as advanced by Charles Darwin, the intelligentsia worldover were amazed at that time. Sri Aurobindo (1872-1950) prophesized that evolution also evolves. With apology to Sri Aurobindo, it may be said that philosophers, particularly when they pronounce a prophesy need not and do not provide any empirical proofs. A literary genius, George Bernard Shaw (1856-1950), wrote a play, *Pygmalion* (1913) and is still being played and displayed in several languages world over. The fantasy involved transformation of a street vending flower-girl to pass on as a princess in 6 months of articulate training in speech and elegant dresses. That was, of course, great entertainment.

But a real life experiment, based on the fundamental conviction of theory of rebirth and reincarnation was put in practice by Annie Besant and Leadbeater. They picked up a destitute boy from a sea beach at Chennai—the then Madras. The boy is a legend today in the form of J. Krishnamurthy (1895-1986). He transformed numerous lives. This transformation of J. Krishnamurthy is a living proof that not only the miracles still happen but, a miracle may also be brought about!

We derive further strength to our logic by citing a few excerpts from yet another poem by Sri Aurobindo.

The Dwarf Napoleon

Behold, by Maya's fantasy of will
A violent miracle takes sudden birth,
The real grows one with the incredible.
In the control of her magician wand
The small achieves things great, the base things grand.

> This puny creature would bestride the earth
> Even as the immense colossus of the past.
> Napoleon's mind was swift and bold and vast,
> His heart was calm and stormy like the sea,
> His will dynamic in its grip and clasp.
> His eye could hold a world within its grasp
> And see the great and small things sovereignly……

We cite excerpts from yet another poem by Sri Aurobindo where a dwarf—a small occurrence of a dwarf human being advances to gigantic dimensions.

> **A Dream of Surreal Science**
>
> A thyroid, meditating almost nude
> Under the Bo-tree, saw the eternal Light
> And, rising from its mighty solitude,
> Spoke of the Wheel and eightfold Path all right……

The poems are cited for their inspirational qualities. If one were to think of Napoleon, one should also remember that he met his Waterloo. However, it may have happened that, "Meditator under a Bo-tree" may have guided subtly. During the period of the stem cell work, we were closely connected with the Dalai Lama. Fourfold expression of this connection in the form of Amitabh, Avlokiteshwar, Ratnasambhava and Amoghasiddhi Buddha including the feminine form Tara have been the symbols for our meditation in this journey. We trust they were really the mentors beyond all mentors to guide.

Our study of anatomy did inspire a lot of awe and respect for the design of the form. Intricate design of structures and organs within the body must have been crafted by some superhuman being. The rhythmic function of physiology so as to automatically correct any dysfunction within a specified limit would defy even cybernetic auto-corrections by a super-computer. Even when pathology professors and authors of textbooks such as William Boyd, with a great flourish of language were warning not to see any teleological design in the process of inflammation, where white blood corpuscles will migrate to the required site and would like to term the process as Chemotaxis—a process mediated only because of the shift of molecules—it was difficult for us not to ask, but who designed chemotaxis?

'Gray's Anatomy' is a work of several geniuses. The book running into over 1200 pages was required to be memorized precisely, particularly if the student was to be a surgeon. The students were provided with some grace whereby the first chapter on The Cell was omitted from study. Thus after having had a successful surgical career extending to even sculpting human body as a plastic surgeon, having discharged a social obligation to the society with more than what I have got from Mother India and having probed even into esoteric realms of states of consciousness, I thought my journey should end now. Fate had other designs for us.

How long would it have been incubated in the subconscious is difficult to guess. But it began in 2004, when I attended the Indian Science Congress at Gandhinagar, Gujarat.

2
Pollution Board Clearance: Ms. Gauri

It must have been around 2004, but it appears to be in the very distant past. Though India is getting more and more clean, it was a different story back then. We were successful in acquiring about two acres of land at Biotech Park, Savli, Vadodara. The dream of building a stem cell laboratory was ambitious.

The first requirement was to get a clearance from Pollution Control Board. British left Independent India, fermenting with fierce idealism by a few and an utterly dirty country. Dirty habits and dirty mentality from a huge mass of populace apart, we have accepted physical dirt as nothing unusual.

A change in attitude was first noticed by us when Fritj of Capra sat for an hour with the then Prime Minister, Indira Gandhi. Within that hour Capra sensed uncommon wisdom in the personage of Iron Lady of India. Indira Gandhi also derived some further common sense that Independent India needed clean air, water and forests. There was no Uncommon Wisdom to this; it is elementary. So a new ministry to administer this came to be established.

As per the norms laid down by this ministry, each and every new industry was required to have a clearance from Regional Pollution Control Board. Our scientists got hold of the blank application forms. I decided to submit the form personally. An appointment was promptly granted. I used to wear white, plain *Khadi* at that time. The officer gave me a quick head to toe screening look. He nodded his head sideways a few times, I did not understand anything and sat down.

The pollution control officer called two of his subordinates and said: Our Chief Minister has a wide vision. He has, therefore, set up a Biotechnology Park, the applicant, Dr. Vyas here is the first one to be allotted a slot at the park and he is the first one to approach us for clearance. He has already liaisoned with an agency to clear various kinds of waste materials and chemicals. I propose that we grant permission to proceed. Would you both agree?

In silent agreement, the subordinates signed at the marked spots. We were told that the application will be forwarded to the head office at Gandhinagar, we should soon hear from them.

Yes, it was true that we heard from the head office in a short time. There were no mobile phones then, only landlines. A voice identifying himself as an officer of Pollution Control Board from Gandhinagar spoke to us. The conversation went thus:

"Am I speaking to Dr. Vyas?"

"Yes."

"I have some interesting propositions for you. We will want to help you by expediting your application."

"Thank you, kindly proceed."

"Yes yes, but please understand that the protocol has to be followed."

"Please follow the protocol expeditiously, we shall be obliged."

"No no, Dr. Vyas please understand. The protocol is about understanding *Vyavahar*."

I said with some consternation, "I do not understand *Vyavahar*. Please explain."

"Do not be so naïve, Dr. Vyas", the voice said coyly. "When you are about to embark on a business, you would have known how business is conducted with bureaucrats and the government. Our ministers also understand *Vyavahar*."

"Sorry but I do not understand what *Vyavahar* is."

Now the voice at the other end turned the tenor. "Well, if you are so stubborn as not to understand, then, believe me, you may have to wait for many long long years. The cost of the project will escalate...."

"Sir, leave the cost, etc. to me and I put the phone down." I was fuming internally. What a fall, my countrymen!

Setting our first feet on Biotechnology platform, we had decoded the genetic code in Rabindranath Tagore's poem:

Where the mind is without fear and the head held high;
Where knowledge is free;
Where the world has not been broken up into fragments by narrow domestic walls;
Where words come out from the depth of truth;
Where tireless striving stretches its arms towards perfection;
Where the clear stream of reason has not lost its way into the dreary desert sand of dead habit;
Where the mind is led forward by Thee into ever-widening thought and action;
Into that heaven of freedom, my Father, let my country awake.

I was emotionally propelled with indignation. I found the secretary, Ms. Gauri, who was in-charge of the Board. Her secretary immediately connected me when I disclosed the agenda as 'reporting corruption'. I described the conversation verbatim to her. She asked only one question, "What do you want?", I replied, we want clearance for our project. "Are you sure you don't want to lodge a complaint? And are you not interested in bringing the miscreants to books?"

"No madam, we want to move on with our work."

Late in the evening, Ms. Gauri called up and said, "Your project is cleared. You will get the clearance soon."

I could not believe this. I blurted out, "Ms. Gauri, before you hang up, please tell me, how did this happen?" She replied, "This is business as usual. I called the three officers and asked them who talked to Dr. Vyas today morning? Nobody raised their hand."

She had no sadistic desire to punish the guilty; nor was there any need to educate with a missionary zeal. Our agenda was clearly defined as a request.

"I have seen the proposal. It is entirely in keeping with the requirements. It has been cleared by the local office. I will send over the approval as soon as possible."

She further excused herself, "Dr. Vyas I have to board my flight for Delhi, please excuse me !"

The phone was cut off. There was no time wasted to hear me shout, "Thank you. Thank you so very much!"

That was the last that I have spoken to her. A bureaucrat, honest and efficient bureaucrat, executes elegantly and moves on like the moving finger of Khalil Gibran. I thought of going to Gandhinagar and dropped it because she would consider it to be a waste of her time. Let us hope, in resurgent India, a tribe of bureaucrats like Ms. Gauri flourishes.

3

Dr. H.L. Trivedi – *Bapu*

As I sat down to write the next chapter on the book I got the news about the sad demise of Dr. Hargovind Laxmishanker Trivedi. We studied in the same class at medical college, Ahmedabad. He came to be known amongst his friends as *Bapu.* This was because he was really large hearted. He generously shared his notes and knowledge with his friends including examination tips. He would even forgive the examiner who asked him to repeat, by an explanation that he could not explain the facts for better understanding.

We needed to learn the first few protocols on stem cell research. When I called him in 2004 to ask for an appointment to meet, it was with considerable difficulty that I could get him on line. When I identified myself in English, he immediately reverted back in Gujarati. And thereafter I never had to wait for him to come on the line.

At the meeting I explained my ambitious plans to float a company with dedicated research to stem cells. He was modest. He said he will surely share what he has. This was just after the time that he became famous for having treated the first juvenile diabetes patient! He introduced me to Dr. Aruna Vanikar. Dr. Aruna showed me around their lab. She showed me the book of protocols at their lab and when I asked for the copy she provided it without hesitation. I was rather surprised by the spontaneity and, asked do you not want to patent your protocols? Her reply was, you are recommended by Dr. Trivedi and moreover our philosophy is that knowledge gets larger when we share. They also agreed to train one of our scientist without any fees.

H.L. Trivedi was much ahead of his times. When he presented his work demonstrating how Mesenchymal stem cells will protect a failing kidney, most of the people in the audience did not believe him. His lofty aim was to produce a nephron from stem cells. This I was reminded when a stem cell researcher from Oxford approached us for a placement with the ambition that he expects to create a nephron, citing Dr. Trivedi.

Bapu—Dr. H.L. Trivedi deserved much greater eminence and he would have got it had he continued to work in Canada. He instinctively returned to serve India and this has now been recognised posthumously by the Prime Minister Narendra Modi.

4
National Science Congress: Professor Balu

Almost all stem cell science students in their innocent naivety would have dreamt of producing a clone—a complete organism. It can be elegantly argued that if an embryonic, pluripotent stem cell can give rise to a full human form in uterus, it can certainly do so provided an environment needed for an embryo in uterus can be created in a lab. Elegance of such logic will provide the first proof that this is indeed plausible.

Such happenings would occur only when the mind is overflowing with joy. Beautiful ideas would be full at brim when they are true. Aesthetic idea, even in hard core science would eventually fructify as truth. Let us derive a further substance to the argument as evidenced from a conversation recorded with Nobel Laureate, Paul Dirac, a professor of theoretical physics.

"*Questioner*: Prof. Dirac, your work is on quantum mechanics and quantum electrodynamics. Does it not amount to a mere abstraction?

Dirac: No, there are mathematical proofs.

Questioner: But there is no experiment, no empirical evidence in an experimental laboratory. And the mathematics is only on paper. How do you verify your theory?

Dirac: Yes, my work begins with mathematical equations on paper. I only need a paper and a pencil. But, when everything flows with perfect elegance, I know that this theory is most likely to be true. Elegance, beauty, aesthetics and truth are interwoven."

With this state of mind, I started demurring about the phenomena of a single clone. The sheep 'Dolly' will live for eternity in history as the first and last clone produced out of a stem cell created from a somatic cell. Dolly was cloned by somatic cell nucleus transplantation technique. The nucleus from the ova of the donor sheep was transferred to the udder cell of the recipient sheep cell and was put in the surrogate sheep which gave rise to first sheep clone 'Dolly.' This experiment was done in Scotland in 1996.

'Dolly' suffered from joint problems all over her body. The sheep died after a short life due to lung problems, however, cloning is now banned across the world. This is because in spite of being a pinnacle of scientific achievements, such research was a clear violation of time honoured ethics. There was an outrage from the Church. It certainly threatened the future of humanity. Yet, every stem cell researcher will like to bask in the glory of such a creation.

Towards the end of the twentieth century, another kind of stem cell research that drew worldwide attention was for the treatment of Parkinson's disease. The most potent stem cell is embryonic stem cell. This cell has properties to regenerate into any of the organs. Embryonic cells derived from aborted fetuses were used in the research to develop a treatment from Parkinson's disease. Though it worked, it was a clear violation of ethics. The then President of USA, personally a devout catholic banned stem cell research all together. This was like throwing the baby out with the bath water.

The next President, Barack Obama was petitioned by some 34 top stem cell scientists that they will move out to Europe unless this decision was revoked. Barack Obama lifted the ban arguing thus: "Science, Research and the laboratories have endless patience but a patient cannot wait. His life is threatened and his time is limited. Benefits of cutting edge science research are his prerogative to ask for and should not be denied."

India also put Stem cell research as a funding priority. And, with this kind of atmosphere an entire day was devoted at National Science Congress, 2005 at Ahmedabad, Gujarat.

We met Dr. Noshir Antia at the session. (He was the first Indian to be trained in plastic surgery by A.B. Wallace at Edinburgh; I was the last Indian to be trained by Mr. Wallace). It was a pleasure to sit next to him to listen to some "cutting edge science research" about stem cells.

I asked him, "What are you doing here?"

He said, "Learning about stem cells".

I asked, "Learning, at your age? About stem cells?"

Dr. Antia sat through the session till the lunch break !

It was inspiring to see someone of his seniority still eager and keen to learn.

Although, overall there was a paucity of basic science research presentations, there was some compensation when Dr. Dorairajan Balasubramanian delivered his presentation on stem cells from the limbus. Limbus is a junctional area between sclera and cornea that is studded with stem cells. In normal life the limbal cells constantly keep regenerating the cornea.

At the onset, the speaker provided some humour by announcing that his name is wrongly spelled. He should be named simply "Balu". And at the end he introduced his protégé, a young ophthalmologist, Virendra Sangwan. He had salvaged many eyes by using limbal stem cells. Thus even a corneoplasty was not warranted.

I met Virendra Sangwan several times thereafter. We visited him at L.V. Prasad Eye Institute in Hyderabad. Professor Balu and Virendra were extremely humble and graciously gave us a tour of their stem cell laboratory. They further introduced us to their gentle stem cell scientist, Gita Vemuganthy.

Looking at their laboratory we were struck as to how simple the design of the laboratory was. Immediately in our mind we could see that we could reproduce a stem cell laboratory at Vadodara. There were no anterooms to the laboratory, there was no changing of the dress and a few scientists including Dr. Gita were in simple white coat aprons.

Dr. Gita introduced us to an inverted microscope. I confess that till this date we had not seen an inverted microscope !

We asked Dr. Gita, "Why do you call it inverted?"

She replied, "Because the objectives of the microscope are under the stage (unlike the normal light microscope) and light source is over the stage."

Like a school boy I asked, "But then how can object be viewed if it is under the stage."

She replied, "When you look into the eyepiece you see the object to be viewed. That is the arrangement."

And half jokingly and half serious asked, "Have you come to LVP to see some stem cells or understand how does an inverted microscope work?"

She showed us Limbal stem cells in the initial stage following harvest from the limbal region of the donor eye. She further showed us how after culture the cells come together to form a membrane akin to the cornea.

Dr. Gita told us her story of how she came to be involved in stem cell research. To begin with she was a child specialist. Then she converted herself to a pathologist. The third generation as a stem cell scientist came about due to a transformation by Prof. Balu.

On the stem cell platform she had advanced by leaps and bounds and had travelled the world. She had conducted several workshops to teach prospective scientists about limbal stem cells.

Imagine out surprise when a few years later, Gita wrote us a sad, sentimental farewell letter. She wrote that she was leaving stem cell science with a heavy heart since she had been offered deanship at a medical college. What a loss to the cause of advancing science !

A few years later we wrote to her about the possibility of researching stem cells for regenerating retina in a blind eye. Regrettably she would neither accept to be a part of the project nor could she find a way to facilitate us.

Strange are the ways that people in various situations assigning value to their work. To our esteem, Gita was on the peak sublime, so why would she have agreed to the ridiculous domain of administration? Maybe there was a clash of egos?

Let me talk about our dealings with various scientists at the National Centre for Cell Biology, Hyderabad.

Dr. Balu was the head of the institute who was succeeded by Dr. Lalji, both eminent biotechnologists. After retiring from the NCCB, Dr. Balu became mentor at L.V. Prasad Eye Institute in Hyderabad. We had planned to approach Dr. Lalji with a plan to see if he and Dr. Balu both could work with us together on a project. We were forewarned, that if you mention Dr. Balu's name, then there would be no collaboration with the NCCP.

We accepted that prejudices prevail in the scientific world. We decided that we will try and recruit both of them to help without mentioning one to the other.

We also met a cell scientist at NCCB who was a cardiothoracic surgeon. He asked us, "Do you want to repeat the mistake that I have done?"

We understood what he meant. It was an abject admission of a mistake to change his career from clinical to laboratory research. There was no point in discussing his mistakes. We requested him to take us to the science laboratory. We understood that laboratory research is painstaking slow and rewards are difficult to accrue. We also have collaborated with one further cell biologist at NCCB, Hyderabad. To start with, we will like not name him. Vatsal suddenly looked at me and stopped transcribing.

He asked, "We have been mentioning most people by name, why do we not mention him?"

I answered, "The situation changes to a different paradigm when the relationships between the subordinates and the superiors are concerned, particularly in a government job."

"What is the shift? I do not understand."

"In such a situation, organizational behaviour gets so complex that it becomes archetypal. Are you familiar with archetypal relationships in a Hindu family, such as mother-in-law and daughter-in-law relationships?"

"But that was the mentality which is fast vanishing in modern society."

"Yes, it will be a good evolution for the families and the societies. Few decades ago a British historian and author Parkinson wrote Parkinson's Law. He became famous by articulately defining the relationship between a subordinate and a superior officer. Simply stated, it can be said to be an existence between a dog and a cat or between a cat and a mouse. The law states that there is a spontaneous, inbuilt jealousy between the first and the second rank in the hierarchy everywhere."

"The relevance of not mentioning this brilliant cell biologist by name lies in the fact that we did not want him to suffer by inviting the ire of his superior."

On our first interaction with this cell biologist, he asked,

"Dr. Vyas, how many patients would you have benefited so far?"

"Difficult to count. Innumerable."

"And the patients have now stopped coming to you?"

"When we decided to quit clinical practice, our hospital was overflowing."

"Have you killed any patient?"

"No. But some did die under our treatment."

"Of course that can be understood."

"But let me summarize that I have killed numerous mice and other animals. This was with the hope that my research may ultimately benefit the patients."

"What has happened as of now is that I have a prestigious position at a national institute. It has allowed me to live and nurture my family—this is the only benefit accrued to me by this position. I would be happy to give you the entire protocol to use for patients who need it, say burns and such other injuries."

"That is indeed kind. But, we may not be able to afford it. What would be the approximate cost."

"You will give me happiness, a sense of satisfaction. And no money will change hands." (More details later)

He was true to his word; he collaborated to submit a project for funding under Small Business Innovation Research Initiative (SBIRI). The project was written by him. The project was titled, 'Future potential of the keratinocyte as a somatic cell translating into pluripotent stem cells.'

I decided to send him an email. Vatsal quickly shuffled several screens on the desktop, stopped transcribing and instead sent the following email to this scientist:

'Dear Dr.

Last time we communicated was when you told me about your promotion to a higher authority. You are very much in our memory for your kind courtesy during the visit to NCCB. We wrote a project together as well. Kindly do let us know how you are and what projects are you working on?

With regards,
Bhaskar & Rajni Vyas,
Stem Cell Researchers,
Vadodara.'

By written mail he wrote a reply:

'Dear Sir,

Namaskar. It's a pleasant surprise for me to have received your email. I am very blessed that you remembered me.

I retired from CCMB in April 2017 as Director Grade Scientist. I had been Research Director at Basavatarakam Cancer Hospital and Research Centre for about 2 years.

I am now associated with a start up company (which one of my students started) and involved in producing therapeutic proteins for cancer therapy.

Hope you and all the members in your family are doing well.

Best personal regards
Sridhar.'

He further wrote:

"Basically we are now developing technology to produce immunotherapy drug Pembrolizumab. We have got a World Bank-DBT Grant to do this. As per the projections, we need to keep clone ready for clinical trials by next year. Hopefully we will succeed with blessings from you all.

Secondly, it's a basic and routine protocol that measures cancer cell viability after treatment with any drug. That's the start point."

Thus reconciled that Dr. Sridhar Rao was no more in a subordinate position, we felt comfortable to mention him by his name.

Let me continue the story of our first encounter with him. The cell biologist, Dr. Sridhar Rao Kunchala, explained the elementary difference between a cell and a stem cell. His institution was working on the functions and properties of a cell. His work was focused on cells from the surface of the skin (keratinocytes) of humans and animals. He was working on this cell so as to be able to prepare human skin-like substitute that could be used for treating major skin defects.

My eyes blinked: Eureka!

This was one of my earlier dreams when I had thought of treating my burn patients with cultured keratinocytes. But he explained that this cannot be taken to clinical use because he has not been able to find a substitute for the deeper layer of the skin—dermis. Without this support, the keratinocytes would not survive.

He had spent more than 20 years of his life to develop one cell line. We wondered which way would this dedicated scientist be inferior to Yamanaka who had recently developed a pluripotent stem cell from a skin fibroblast. We understood the answer in our mind. The Indian scientist had the same genius as the Nobel Prize winning Japanese. The difference was not in the seed but in the soil.

We wrote our first project for funding from Government of India in collaboration with Dr. Sridhar Rao. We thought that together we should be able to produce a substitute for human skin. This was to contain a base similar to dermis. Unfortunately, the project was not funded, however it opened a window to approach Professor Padmanabhan that we will narrate in the next chapter.

It is not uncommon for scientist of high eminence to harbour jealousy against colleagues. Vatsal interrupted and said, "But Indian ethos has been different since time immemorial.

Let us study together
Let us eat together, enjoy together
Let us engage in adventure together
So that together we shall excel."

"Yes, this was fundamental to a lifestyle in the times when Krishna and Sudama studied together. It is probable that centuries of alien rule has corrupted this noble idea."

We happened to discuss this incidence with our friends, colleagues and, even the Dalai Lama. In His inimitable style he said, India is our *guru*. A 'chela' that I am, I should not find fault with the *guru*. When further prodded about the Buddhist culture in Japan and the present Indian Hindu ethos, He said imposition of any culture over other is not good. That is the reason why Tibet does not want to be under Chinese domain.

When further questioned, the Dalai Lama expounded thus:

Today, most Japanese are practicing Buddhism. They live by the Buddhist precepts and practice them in real life. Compassion and kindness are basic to Buddhism. Thus conflicts are avoided and may be resolved as well. Avoidance of conflict, even in the mind, saves mental energy. The surplus energy finds its outlet by enhancing creativity.

He was on his fâvourite theme, Buddhist *tantra*. When we continued asking for further elucidation, he initiated us to the formal learning of *Guhya Samaj Tantra*. That was indeed a byproduct of our search for stem cell research. Further discussion is unwarranted here since it will be a distraction from the main story. The dialogue with the Dalai Lama is still in progress encompassing different dimensions that do not include stem cells.

We are now knitting the story once again back to Dr. Balu and stem cells.

The academic gain from the session at "The Indian National Congress of Science" in Gandhinagar was to make the acquaintance with Prof. Balu and Virendra Sangwan. We mused the obituary of A.B. Wallace with Dr. Antia and were about to part when an announcement came. Cadila Pharmaceutical was sponsoring a workshop with two Korean scientists later that evening. Everyone was invited. I darted off and was the first one to register.

I had few other instances when I met Professor Balu. We had no knowledge about the guidelines for stem cell research. Gujarat State Biotechnology Mission (GSBTM) invited all stem cell researchers and scientists from Gujarat to discuss the scenario and academics regarding stem cells. Professor Balu was in Chair. He made an oblique remark without mentioning Dr. H.L. Trivedi. He said, "I am told that there are some fly by night scientist in Gujarat etc." I protested that there are no fly by night scientists—they have done a yeomen's service to humanity. But worst was still to come when a scientist sitting next to me was asked to describe what he is working on. Dr. Himanshu Patel started describing how he has produced myocardial cells from stem cells and help treat 78 cardiac patients in cardiac failure. He had barely finished when Professor Balu flared up. "So here is fly by night stem cell scientist." He lambasted Dr. Himanshu and proceeded to tear him to pieces I had to intervene.

I said "Dr. Balu, if a scientist has helped 78 cardiac patients with a fastidious process like culturing myocardial cells, and published his work; kindly tell us what is so fly by night about this?"

I had forgotten that I was speaking to one of the highest authorities in India in the scientific field. Probably this might have been for the first time that Prof. Balu would have been accosted thus by a novice. Everyone was stunned. After some silence Dr. Balu said yes there may not be anything wrong. But the regulations have not been followed.

Thereafter, we had made a permanent friend with Dr. Himanshu Patel. However, Prof. Balu was correct; *not* on scientific grounds but *on legal terms.* A detailed discussion is warranted on the subject that had profound implications on our work and our future, we shall talk about it later. A few times after this incidence when our paths crossed with Dr. Balu on scientific terms, we greeted him with high regards. He has made immense contributions by becoming a mentor to L.V. Prasad Eye Institute including sourcing a even confocal microscope for the institute. He has cordially reciprocated my greeting by an informal, 'Hi Bhaskar!'

We have decided to focus on what is good and turn a blind eye to what is sordid. Regulations are needed for all kinds of activities and a good government with good governance without any corruption is the primary need to regulate. We reiterate and dare to say that stem cell therapy is futuristic. Even when a single spinal cord injury or amyotropic lateral sclerosis of spinal cord patient benefited so as to live a productive life with stem cell therapy, further advancement of research is warranted. Alas! The regulations in India are drafted—crafted with a copy and paste of 'advanced nations', primarily FDA, USA. National newspapers including *The Hindu* gave front page coverage that a stem cell researcher-medical doctor may be punished with a revocation of his medical licence and imprisonment of up to 2 years if they did not adhere to the rules laid down by the

Government of India! Even Virendra Sangwan, a profulgent pioneer of limbal stem cell research, a protégé of Prof. Balu that received the Rashtrapati Award for best young scientist of the year, was forced to admit that he had not conducted any clinical trials. It seems history repeats itself—under the threat of execution by the Church, even Galileo had to admit that the earth was flat!

The current corona virus pandemic has forced a radical rethink in how new drugs and vaccines are brought into clinical use. Numerous drug trials have been on fast track the world over and the race to produce a new vaccine is promised to bring it to the front-line within months rather than years.

5
Indravadan Modi

We had known Indravadan Bhai some 50 years ago. He had founded Cadila, a pharmaceutical company in early 1960s. It was in a small building in the Ellisbridge area (Ahemadabad). One can imagine him cycling to and fro Ellisbridge with a couple of bags full of samples for budding doctors that including myself. His story is the success story of a hard working first generation successful entrepreneur in post-independence India.

Cadila sponsored a workshop with 2 Korean researchers at the science conference in Gandhinagar in 2004. They were invited by Cadila Company to lecture and demonstrate on their success stories about stem cell applications. The post-congress workshop went on till early morning next day.

We asked one of the volunteers as to how much would Cadila have spent to sponsor this workshop?

He answered, "Peanuts for Cadila."

With surprise we asked: even after sponsoring the two Korean presenters?

"You do not know what Cadila is today."

The brilliant Korean stem cell scientists showed their breath taking research. We saw for the first time myocardial cells pulsating in a petri dish that were obtained with translation. (This was the secret that they did not want to reveal. They did not describe the source and the method of translation). They also showed to everyone's astonishment regeneration from spinal cord injury. When a paralysed person is shown to be walking after few months, with the help of stem cell treatments, who would not like to develop this kind of technology? Korean presenters emphasised on multilateral collaborations. Their emphasis was on multidisciplinary approach. They were humble to acknowledge that the team would comprise several researchers. Total number of collaborators amounted to about 2 dozens.

As clinicians, they happened to deliver the products to the patient. And therefore, the limelight in which they are basking is primarily not their own entirely but a sum total of several hands and multiple brains working together. They distributed their contact details and said they would be happy to answer more details by email.

They did not answer any academic questions that I was naïve enough to ask. Cutting edge research in biotechnology would have cost them a fortune. We, the medical doctors, take pride in showing and teaching our expertise. That is a different domain from innovations. We had hardly known about patents at that time. Now it seems elementary that why did they not answer though initially volunteered by them. Had there been a business proposal from Cadila or someone that was capable of buying their research, someone from their team would have certainly answered with a business proposal. And the academics would have been the last to be disclosed.

We returned to Vadodara with a firm resolve. We decided to dedicate ourselves to stem cell research. I stopped operating. Rajni stopped registering further patients for delivery. Operating room was converted to a stem cell laboratory. We had not thought of following any particular kind of business model. But surely we knew that Government of India was funding biotechnology research. It was imperative that, to avail this funding, the applicant must be a registered private limited company. We registered a company and called it Total Potential cells.

We decided to pay our respects to Indravadan bhai, since he was the motivator. Writing from his personal email id, he asked us to come over to Bhat once again. Graciously he sent his car to pick us up from the station… At the reception, a gentleman approached us and shook our hands.

"I am Dr. P.K. Ghosh."

"Nice to meet you, we have come to meet Indravadan Bhai."

"Yes you are welcome."

"Are you a stem cell scientist?"

"No, I am a fellow of Royal Society. Are you F.R.C.S. ?"

"No. I am happy with a single degree. Master of Surgery."

"But you were in England?"

"Yes. And I had spent another year in USA as well."

"What did you do in the laboratory over there with Dr. John Howard?"

I understood that Dr. Ghosh had previewed our biodata.

He spent a leisurely half an hour discussing some of the aspects of stem cell science. We told him how delicate the stem cells are. They get easily infected. And the entire culture is lost. Further I was required to explain to him how an over-growth of stem cells can also be detrimental and cause apoptosis. Apoptosis is massive death when the cells over-grow. Apoptosis was being discussed in media that year since the three researchers were jointly awarded a Nobel Prize for this discovery. The lay press called it, 'Kiss of Death'. I tried to make the conversation light by adding that the three Nobel Laureates to be survived by sharing the prize because they were continents apart working in different laboratories. At this time Dr. Ghosh got up.

We did not understand, so I blurted, "Dr. Ghosh, but we were here to see Indravadan Bhai."

"Yes. Yes. He will see you soon" and left.

He came to call us after a few minutes. He seemed to be happy. Indravadan Bhai was sitting with a medical doctor, an ophthalmologist, Bakulesh Khamar. He asked, "You want to change your career as a researcher in stem cells? Why? There was not enough money and…." he laughed.

"Indravadan Bhai, we Gujaratis value money, but we are satisfied that we have enough to live on. We thank you for providing highly useful academic information on what stem cell science holds for the future."

"When was that?", he asked.

"At the last day of National Science Congress and also thereafter listening to the Korean researchers that you sponsored."

Looking at Dr. Ghosh he asked, "How much would it cost to set up a laboratory for these doctors?"

Ghosh quickly calculated and replied, "38 lakhs".

"And do we have enough space?"

"Yes."

Indravadan Bhai extended his hand and said, "Dr. Vyas we will give you 38 lakh. Set up the laboratory. Do research leisurely and swim in the swimming pool when you like. Talk to me once in a while."

I was taken aback. Astonished. I had not expected, asked or even indicated a need for money. Holding his hand, I pressed it hard and I blurted out, "Indravadan Bhai thank you, thank you so very much. But our purpose was to convey our gratitude for doing what you did for the furtherance of stem cell research. We were provided motivation, that is what we really needed but we have not come to ask for any money. Thank You."

Indravadan Bhai dropped his hand.

There is a story about the benign innocence of a saint Dionysus. He was sitting in sunshine on a rock when Napoleon approached him riding on a horse. Two men, belonging to altogether different walks of life had a fruitful dialogue. Napoleon seemed to have benefited and asked the saint to ask for a favour. Dionysus is said to have asked for the return of sunshine since Napoleon had blocked it with him riding on the horse.

My response was archetypal, since I had adored this story since my adolescence. As we were born in pre-independence era, we were taught to guard our self-respect from the British and the response came as a conditioned reflex. I had little known about the large-heartedness and nationalist personality of Shri Indravadan Bhai. In promoting his brand, he campaigned against 'Angreji Dawa' thereby refuting the then prevalent multinational companies. Here was a start-up that had not even started work in his company, talking to a self made, builder of a pharmaceutical empire. We should have known better as to how to be courteous in declining his offer.

The norms for productive and constructive behaviour in the twenty first century demand that co-operation and coalition should prevail. The giver and the taker both have different needs and in the quest for the fulfilment of their needs, they collate. Indravadan Bhai is no more now. Had he been there we would have paid him one more visit apologise for my behaviour on that day.

Dr. Ghosh came out and before parting he sat with us for some more time again. He said that a patent has expired for Monoclonal antibodies. There is huge market worldwide. He would like to be a partner with us in developing this product. We simply asked, "What are monoclonal antibodies? We do not know."

Dr. Ghosh remains a long time friend. But we now understand how not to be so naïve as to not understand the generosity of a large hearted person or offer for collaboration from a highly placed (we came to know later that P.K. Ghosh was Vice President, Cadila Pharmaceuticals) scientist.

We were offered a return journey in a brand new "Rolls Royce" car.

Musing over this incidence with some regret, we derived some wisdom. Stem cell research is an expensive endeavour. This was better understood by our friends than us. Since this encounter we have received generous help from numerous well-wishers; they never posed to be condescending. We remain ever grateful for their generosity.

6
Gentleman Vishnu Varshney: A Blessing from Saibaba

We have lived the prime time of our life in a close fisted pseudo-socialist economy in India. Following liberation and globalization, we learnt new terminologies such as angel investors, venture capital funding, etc. We doubted the existence of such entities. My daughter Nirupa (A MBA in finance and a doctorate in the share market), verified that, not only are they operative in Gujarat and India, but they succeed as well.

Hence we decided to approach Gujarat Venture Finance Limited at Ahmedabad.

Within a few days, I received a phone call. The caller said, "Dr. Vyas, I am the official in-charge of finances at GVFL. I would like to speak regarding your proposal. Would you kindly keep our talk anonymous?" With a pleasant surprise, I said, "Yes, of course. Please speak."

"I am aware about the potential benefits of stem cell therapy. My new born baby boy had a birth defect. He is alive and progressing following stem cell therapy. I have spoken to Mr. Varshney about this. So he is suitably inclined to fund your venture. He is likely to call for a presentation soon."

"That is splendid, we will meet you then."

"I have moved for a better position elsewhere and I am being relieved today. Best of luck to your efforts."

So here was a guardian angel, materializing from nowhere! I

said to myself, "If a guardian angel has spoken, surely there will be angel investors as well!"

I had to move fast, I realized. I wrote down the cheque towards payment of the plot for Biotech Park, Savli and started making a presentation together with Rajni and other members of my team. We have presented academic research at the conferences pertaining to our medical subjects. This was an entirely different challenge.

This was, however, our first ever presentation on stem cells. Moreover we had prepared highly optimistic visions of what would happen in 2010, 2020 etc. for smaller informal presentations on stem cells. We had absolutely no idea about how to present to potential investors whose primary aim was to generate a profit from this proposal. We were invited to present to Mr. Varshney at Ahmedabad.

The first projected slide read as thus: 'Survival of the fittest'.

Survival of the fittest or the adaptable

To accommodate, to adjust, to fit, to accept — concession or yielding
Survival strategy — in response to physiological or pathological demands
Adapt — to conform to changes in environment — internal and external
Most cells have the inherent plasticity—

Vishnu Varshney stopped us rightaway; he said "Please be specific. We do not like to have multiple colours and disjointed statements. Tell us about what you wish to do with your products."

We skipped several slides and projected the next one.

Drug Discovery—"There are many reasons to be interested in stem cells, one of the most prominent being their use in finding better drugs to treat human diseases. This presentation focuses on how this may be implemented. Recent advances in the production of reprogrammed adult cells and their regulated differentiation to disease-relevant cells are the products, and diseases that have been modelled using these methods are discussed."

Varshney nodded, "This is a little better. Move forward."

Avoiding the academic distinctions between the varieties of stem cells, we focused on the limbal stem cells from the junction of sclera and cornea to benefit patients with corneal defects, how the stem cells will be converted into myocardial cells that can benefit a patient with heart failure and how a stem cell transforms into a nerve cell which can benefit a neurological patient.

Varshney asked, "Do you mean that such a cell can help a brain stroke patient?"

"Yes, there is enormous literature in support. But in India so far there are no clinical trials."

"And what about spinal cord injuries?"

"Korean scientists have demonstrated the beneficial results of stem cell transplantation in patients with spinal cord injuries."

"What would you say about a baby born with meningocele?"

I paused and wondered, did the baby mentioned by the finance manager on the phone have such a defect?

"There are several grades to this condition. And we do not know the status of stem cell with them."

We presented the project cost estimate at Rs. 10 crore.

When we concluded our presentations, Vishnu Varshney began his comments:

Your project is well articulated academic study but it is highly ambitious.

We will advise you to restrict your research to a single product that can be taken to commercialization as soon as possible. It may take about 3 years and your projection to yield profit in a year or so is ill-founded.

I could not hide my disappointment. I did not utter a word but gave up a deep sigh. Varshney saw my body language and said:

"GVFL not only funds a start-up, we shall become your stakeholders and will provide a mentorship too in the domains that you will need for sure, such as marketing, business promotion and future expansion."

... You have hurried up to acquire a large area of land at Biotech Park that is not necessary for a start-up but we will take this on our books. I thought what is the next missile that he is going to aim to me? Fortunately it came as a bulldozer creating a pavement erasing an obstacle…. "Your project estimate is Rs. 10 crore. That also is not needed for a start-up. GVFL does not have much money. Your total funding requirement is Rs. 10 crore out of which GVFL will like to fund you with Rs. 2 crore!"

I could not believe my ears! I got up and extended my hand with a few steps forward towards Vishnu Varshney and said "Bhagwaan Vishnu, you are our truly incarnate Bhagwaan. Thank you, thank you very much!"

He dismissed his team and asked our assistants also to leave. Thereafter he switched over to an informal friendly mode. In a relaxed easy-chair, he almost rumbled in a monologue as how he learnt about the concept of a venture fund in USA. How he was the first one in India to bring the concept to Gujarat. With what difficulties he could barely pursue the existing profit making business houses to participate in raising equity so that GVFL can be incorporated. His estimate was that if 3 out of 10 funded start-up companies would succeed, that would be enough for GVFL to keep afloat. 7 out of 10 funded companies by GVFL are profit making. He also gifted us a few books written by him regarding venture funding. At this time, one of our team members entered and reminded that we had to catch a train from Vadodara to go to Bombay that evening.

But Bhagwaan Vishnu laid down a totally unexpected condition. He said, "I am a firm believer that the entire cosmos is governed by divine forces. I further believe that Satya Saibaba of Shirdi, though not in physical form now, is still functioning as an arbitrator so that the divine grace accrues only for the benefit of large masses of people. His benevolence so ordains that the Divine Grace descends only in the right direction. It can never do any harm."

"Yes, Mr. Varshney, we are firm believers in your philosophy. We had a pilgrimage along with our daughters to the shrine at Shirdi."

"Oh, and what did Sai tell you? To go to Vishnu Varshney?"

"We spent one night at the shrine, we hoped that the fabled Saibaba does give *Darshan* in the early morning in the courtyard of the temple. We got up at 3:30 A.M. and in the courtyard, we saw numerous other people, aspiring with the same motivation. We waited till dawn, the crowd started dispersing. We also made our way to a tea stall with a thought that Sai may have found more worthy people than us to bless. Or he may have thought that we may also be satisfied that he has already blessed us. Though our selfish wish to see an evidence, may be rather obscure in the form of an apparition of Sai Baba moving around blessing the devotees."

"Saibaba did not speak to us, but maybe he prodded in our unconscious domain to approach you and GVFL."

"Okay then, I have put up a small shrine of Saibaba in the extreme western end of the hall, go and ask for his blessing. I repeat this has to be done if you wish that you will benefit with your association with GVFL."

Hurriedly we rushed to the small, elegantly decorated shrine, pledged our obeisance and left GVFL and Ahmedabad driving at a crazy speed of 100 km/h. With or without our knowledge, maybe Saibaba protected us on the highway and we made it to the train with seconds to spare.

My mind was neither on the highway nor with the dangers of the speed. I was absorbed about how the blessings from Saibaba will descend and, with an axiomatic query that "Is Saibaba god? And if so, where does God exist, etc."

Apparitions have been a subject of our wonder and disbelief, but given to argue on both sides and having read the stories narrated by Dilip Kumar Roy such as his works as 'Amongst the Great' and 'Miracles Still Happen', we keep on searching and have not given up. In the course, we came across a spiritual person at Theosophical Society, Chennai. We narrate the story that he told in 1st person narrative. He asked,

"Do you believe in God?"

"I do and I do not, it depends upon circumstances."

"I was a confirmed atheist to myself and to the rest of the world and I confirmed that God, you do not exist, so I don't believe in you."

"I was standing on a high cliff of Alps Mountains and my foot slipped. I happened to fall. At that time I shouted, 'God, I do believe in you now, I cry for help and please help!' at that time my hands came to clutch upon a root jutting out of a cliff and I stopped falling."

I continued to shout, "God even when I told you that I now believe in you and asked for help. But you do not exist, so how would you have helped me? I let go the root that my hands were holding.

Continued to fall when I heard God shouting back to me, "My dear devotee, the root that you were holding was my hand!" The rest of the story is for all of us to believe or not believe but surely to have a good laugh.

How is a belief generates the physiological changes in a human being is articulately worked out by Bruce Lipton in his treatise on Biology of Belief. But we have probed deeper into about how the domain of a human brain connects to the universe. Intense meditative thought is the creative power of thought. How the creative power of thought cannot be explained even with the equation propounded by Einstein: $e = MC^2$ *is well known…* But it may take a long time to exactly decipher the mechanism of transfer of creative power of thought to formative facilitation into material realization of visualization. We believe that visualization should be practiced again and again to generate and strengthen formative facilitation. This is how creative power happens.

Idea is the first reality. Atom bombs that exploded at Hiroshima and Nagasaki are empirical evidences on a massive scale. This real life story of stem cell is also a miniscule of empirical evidence of this fact.

At this juncture of transcription, Vatsal invoked Epicurus. And Epicurus started speaking thus:

> *"Is God willing to prevent evil, but not able? Then he is not omnipotent.*
> *Is he able, but not willing? Then he is not malevolent.*
> *Is he both able and willing? Then whence cometh evil?*
> *Is he neither able nor willing? Then why call him God?"*

At this instant Nietzsche shouted: "Yes there is no need. God is dead." Thus spoke Zarathustra repeatedly in four volumes. However, Einstein resurrected God a few decades later with a public dialogue with Neil Bohr proclaiming,

Einstein: Quantum theory is probabilistic. I cannot believe that God is playing dice with the universe.

Neil Bohr: Einstein, leave the God to do his work. As physicists, let us carry on with our work founded on sound mathematical equations.

Here Stephen Hawking interjected: I can prove that there is a divine design utilizing Newtonian physics only: On the contrary with elegant equations I can also prove that probabilities do exist and the outcome is determined simply by a chance observation.

This multiple dialogue can go on probably till eternity and still the choice will have to be individually since there will be no conclusion. But this will stray us away from our limited agenda of Saibaba's blessings *vis-à-vis* funding by GVFL.

Vishnu Varshney kept his word. A few days later, he visited our premises with a professor of pharmacology, Dr. Harish Padh, a biotechnologist working as Director of B.V. Patel Pharmaceutical Education and Research Development Centre. Varshney introduced Prof. Padh and said he would assess our research capabilities for further innovations.

When I summarized my published papers, more than 30, pertaining to surgical procedures and my innovative surgical practices, Prof. Padh simply nodded his head. Obviously he was not interested. But when Rajni talked about her publications, his face lit up when she talked about her concept of psychodynamics of unexplained reproductive failure. Her paper had used a modified Huener's test which was published as Vyas' Modification. Psychotherapeutic treatment to combat the immunosuppression at the cervix had succeeded in helping couples with unexplained infertility to have children. He asked for the hard copies and immediately reverted back with many thanks and congratulations.

Before leaving our premises to see the allotted plot at Biotech Park, Savli, Varshney approached Rajni and said, "I am impressed. GVFL is interested. I do not lie, I will give you money and I am an honest man. There is no phoney business with Varshney. He talked about two of his proposals; one which he had turned down and another which he had invested in. A lady from Vadodara came with a good proposal but when she talked about the processing cost etc. I shelved her proposal. I was an investor in another company based in Vadodara for a few years. After successful commercial transition to make pure water with reverse osmosis process, I left the company. We will move forward soon, let the Grace of Saibaba prevail."

We went into proactive prospective projections as to how to

deploy Rs. 2 crore. We commissioned an architect to design a laboratory at Biotech Park. We made a list of equipments to be purchased. We listed the alternatives for transport from Vadodara to Biotech Park. Such activities continued for some time when we received a short, terse note from Vishnu Varshney around the time of Janmashtami (Shri Krishna's birthday), thus, GVFL regrets that we will not be able to fund your company. The reasons are as follows:

1. We do not like that you have professorial advisers from the University.
2. The investment in land will be a top-heavy, unnecessary investment.
3. There is a railway crossing that involves delays at the junction with the road. There is too much time wasted.

Firstly, we did not understand that this is a turnabout and a closure. Then agitation and resentment began to mount. This time along with Nirupa, I went to GVFL and absolutely un-business like asked Varshney, "We have seen a gentlemanly Vishnu Varshney, Vishnu the protector deity of the universe. But now probably there would be a thousand names to Bhagwaan Vishnu. How have you come about to the point that you now have become a Ranchchod—deserting us?"

Varshney kept his cool. He would have been justified to ask us to quit. There was no commitment to explain. But in his suave protective ways, he said, "Dr. Vyas, you are a surgeon. I understand that you will not have really known how business gets conducted. Your daughter will understand me for sure, that GVFL is a limited company. There is a board that finally decides the matter. They have to assess the profitability and repayment feasibility." He spent a few minutes talking directly to Nirupa about what transpired at the Board meeting. What were the real objections etc.

Turning at last to me, he said: "You have a qualified talented daughter. Induct her into the company." I was still indignant. Bordering almost to stupidity, obstinately I retorted, "I do not believe in nepotism!"

"No Dr. Vyas, this is being unfair to your own family. But it is your choice."

We drove back to Vadodara, this time leisurely musing to ourselves as to why Saibaba's grace did not descend. Or, was he really unbenevolent executioner of the divine plan so as to dissuade us from an honourous task. Surely the debt has to be paid back, business executed with generation of profits. This had to be done when we were in our 70s. We may have been truly blessed by Saibaba when our selfish projections of ill understood self-interest may not have been granted.

This acceptance of the denial may also be attributed to a neurotic defence. However, we have come to understand that we have learnt to act with courage and conviction and not reflect on the outcome. This has certainly given us stable and lasting friendships whenever we interacted with new people. This is evident by a recently protracted negotiation for a collaboration with a confirmed devotee of Saibaba again, that also crashed. He expressed a sense of guilt for what happened. We wrote back, "We conclude, with profound faith in our scriptures that everything that happens, happens only as an expression of Divine Will; nothing will ever happen without the Grace from the Divine—*Daivam*. Let the Grace of Saibaba prevail."

7
National Science Congress: 2006-07

The Hyderabad Conference in 2006 was held with primary focus on agriculture. Our search for advancement in stem cell science was futile. Even looking for novel ideas in scientific fields, we came across only one presentation that we remember today. It was about an innovative modality to assess sexual stimulation in a male frog by counting the number of times the frog will assume a particular position! A significant gain in the knowledge pool was to make friendship at the first meet with Dr. K. Sridhar Rao. We have discussed the collaboration with Dr. Rao in an earlier chapter.

The next Indian Science Congress was scheduled to be held at Amity University. I attended this Conference alone as Rajni was unable to accompany me. When I started the process of booking my ticket, I came to know that there was a change in venue. It was to be held now at Chidambaram, a small town in South India. Where was this township named Chidambaram ? And how would the change have happened? I took some time to decipher that such a change can only be manoeuvred with all powerful financial arms of the Government of India! The estimated budget for Indian Science Congress that year was INR 75 crore that was to be funded by the Government. The road to the hitherto unknown town Chidambaram passed *via* Pondicherry.

Once again science of stem cell was hardly existent at this Congress as well. But I stumbled upon one more collaborator that was interested in stem cell research. It so happened that I put my hand, rather condescendingly on the shoulder of, who I thought to be a young man who was rushing past and said,

"Young man, take care, you could have fallen."

He replied, "I am Prof. Gopal Kundu. Because of my short stature, I am frequently misunderstood as a post-graduate."

"My apologies, Professor. Where are you working?"

"My lab is at NCCS, Pune. I have half a dozen Ph.D. students working in my lab."

"Oh, I have visited NCCS last year. I met the director to ask facilitation for our stem cell research. Don't you think he is rather conservative?" Little did I realize that this was a wrong question to an immediate subordinate to the director. When I had met the Director G.C. Gupta, he was generous with hospitality but would not even open the conversation about facilitating stem cell research. I had wanted to discuss chondrogeneic translation—(stem cell that got converted into a cartilage producing cell with calcification) from stem cells that were produced by Prof. Vani at NCCS. Even on further nudging, Director Gupta had not obliged. Of course, he had guided me to Prof. Ramesh Bhonde."

Therefore, the expected answer from Dr. Gopal Kundu was, "I invite you to my lab. At that time we will see what is possible."

"When can I come to visit?"

"I am co-sponsoring an international conference at Lonavala, on translational research. Register and come over. I shall be glad to see you there."

This meeting graduated to writing our first funded project for DBT (Department of Biotechnology, India).

However, there was a different dimension that was delivered to us whilst we were at the Congress.

One evening, I decided to drive down to the famous Natraja Temple in Chidambaram. The shrine was so vast that it would have taken me more than a week to study various sculptures and their associated history. What a wonderful panorama it was! I wondered why this temple was not included in one of the most splendorous heritage of mankind! After sitting in awe for a short time when I decided to leave, the chauffeur asked me, "Would you not want to visit Patanjali Cave?" I had not heard of this before and requested him to take me there.

Entering the cave without doors was like the first step of Alice in Wonderland. The cave was like a long, long corridor. On each side of it were rows of lighted oil lamps. I could not venture to go beyond a few steps. And as I sat down, a subtle calmness descended upon me. It was mesmerizing to visualize that in this very cave, Maharshi Patanjali had taught 3000 disciples more than 2 millennia ago! And I started hearing the voice of Maharshi expounding what would he have meant with a short, terse, Sutra: *Ritumbara Pragnya*. With profulgent enlightenment of my own intuitive insight, I realized how a spontaneous generation of *Ashta-Mahasiddhi* would accrue to a meditator! In this moment of timeless experience, I merged with That Alone that Is.

I do not know how long I sat in this experience. A gentle tap on my shoulder brought me back to reality. "It is already getting late and we should reach the venue till the dinner will be served." I acquiesced to his request although I was still basking in the spray of noble thoughts that came cascading like a huge waterfall. That was to provide a genesis of yet another book, 'Space, Time and Consciousness: Rationale of the Paranormal' which is now in its 2nd edition.

I abandoned the morning session the next day that was entirely devoted to discuss Leishmaniasis. This parasitic disease occurs in India, only in the southern region and is unknown to Gujarat and further north. I decided to pay a courtesy call to a professor of anatomy Ramaswamy, who was in his late 70s. Rather than being a courtesy call, it transferred itself into high academics. The professor would have guessed that the aspiring stem cell scientist would not have known some of the marvels that Nature provides in designing the human body. When he asked me at last,

"What is the nerve supply of cornea?"

"Ophthalmic nerve?"

"No."

"Optic Nerve?"

"Optic nerve, second cranial nerve terminates in the retina.

The nerve supply to the cornea is by the ophthalmic branch of 5th cranial nerve. Name the 5th cranial nerve."

"Trigeminal nerve."

"Yes. And is it a myelinated nerve?"(Nerve supplying the sensations to the body structures are provided with a sheath. The sheath is made with a protein structure called myelin.)

"Yes."

"Why do the nerve fibres supplying the cornea not provide opacity to the cornea? I would rather answer than tax you further. Just as the fibres of this branch of myelinated nerves enter transparent structure of cornea, they lose their sheath! What makes the fibres lose myelin? That is the wonder of the Nature. If you believe in God, (which Prof. Ramaswamy and I firmly do), it is God who wants every human being to have a transparent cornea and yet have the sensations as well."

From profound depths of anatomy, he transgressed to his pilgrimage to Amarnath. He then took out a gong from his drawer of his table. He tapped it with a wooden stick. And *Aha*! There came a long reverberating sound of *A*…*u*….*m*… As a parting gift he gave the gong and the stick to me! That still rings and reverberates as a spiritual memory of the professor.

I left Chidambaram treasuring these precious and priceless experiences deep down in my unconscious mind. ***Only to remind once in a while that promises are given and they will be fulfilled***. I spent a day at the Aurobindo Ashram before reaching Chennai Airport. Although the brief had been to understand stem cell research in Chidambaram, I came away with divine experiences that have nourished us both since that time.

8
The Best Beginning is with Zero: Jump into Turbulent Waters

There is a word in Hindi and other Indian languages–*Swabhaav.* I find it difficult to translate the word in English. Deeper probing into semantics of this word may take it to a state whereby the genes responsible for property particular characteristic cannot be deleted. It is an ingrained lifestyle. *Swabhaav* may be decided by culture, family environment, multilateral influences in upbringing and the impact of powerful personalities and for the scientific minded, it by differential gene expression. This is also the subject of current debate—Nature *vs.* Nurture. What was my *Swabhaav* that I jumped into the Ganges at Haridwar in an attempt to swim (much to the consternation of onlookers and causing sheer panic for Rajni and our daughters)? On a much more noble intent what would have inspired us to delve deeper into studying the science of stem cell is an enigma and may require in depth psychoanalysis. And it may still be futile. It is suffice to say that when we decided to do research in stem cell science, our knowledge was at the level 0.

We have referred to *Gray's Anatomy* earlier. The book is a masterpiece that merits to be preserved as a cultural heritage of mankind. And only in 2015, 41st edition of the book has a chapter on stem cells and regenerative medicine, which we continue to read even today! This emphasizes that in learning, repetition and revision are warranted and beginning at 0 will not amount to once again starting at the beginning.

We shut down our multi-speciality hospital that had occupancy of about 120 per cent. Family and friends politely tried to dissuade and some others said at best "utter stupidity!"

We were polite to decline but defiant not to give up. Our motto was derived from Jean Christophe, a hero in Romain Rolland's novel, '*To strive, to struggle; not to find and yet not to yield*.' We said, "I gave up my speciality with a new birth in this life as simply as an inquirer. Associations and specialization are the organs of protection of interests by the concerned groups. Though I would like to remain an evergreen student, if you were to read the names of Nobel Laureates, they have transgressed the narrow confines of their specialization. Stem cells have been studied for more than 100 years and yet there is not a single textbook on the subject."

Study of the chapter on cell biology in *Gray's Anatomy* yielded two collateral benefits—the most wonder of all wondrous discoveries could be said to be the use of Carbon Dioxide in cell culture. Who would not think that it is truly wondrous to know that stem cells need to be cultured in an atmosphere of 5 per cent Carbon Dioxide only!

Discovery of a free radical, Nitric Oxide (NO), sounded almost like 'Eureka!' to us. And the revelation of two other molecules produced with variance in the valency was also a novel discovery to us. We had known Nitrous Oxide as a short term anaesthetic gas. We had known of an accidental death due to mistaken over-usage of this gas instead of oxygen. This had happened during our student days and thereafter, the cylinders of Nitrous Oxide have been differently coloured than Oxygen. However, Nitrogen gas, that constitutes about 80 per cent in ordinary air changes its properties radically in human body, when there is a change in its valency.

Valency is the combining power of an element so that in combination with a negatively charged element it constitutes a molecule. Anaesthetic gas is N_2O. When Nitrogen changes its valency from 4 to 2 it combines with a single Oxygen atom to produce a different kind of gas with amazing properties. This free radical has been playing key roles in transferring information in almost all the cells of the body! This is one of the ways as to how cells talk to each other. It is a signalling molecule involved in many physiological and pathological processes. It can exist in the bloodstream for only a few seconds. Even then, in a short period of time it can produce a cascade of signals.

A similar story, that of the Carbon molecule also produces an *Aha !* experience but in a reverse direction. It is commonplace to understand that carbon dioxide (CO_2) is deleterious and body throws it out with every expiration. Is it not an amazing phenomenon that the best cell culture (multiplication of cells) is obtained using 5 per cent CO_2?

If Carbon was to imitate nitric oxide (NO), carbon monoxide (CO) should also have some similar functions, but we all know that it is more poisonous than carbon dioxide (CO_2). Every inhalation of cigarette smoke does involve a small, miniscule inhalation of carbon monoxide (CO). Injurious effects of smoking are largely attributed to nicotine, but there can be no doubt that a small quantity of CO also contributes to smoking's adverse effects.

Yet another discovery was the fact that feminine sex, ordinarily known as the second sex is biologically untrue. Mitochondria are the powerhouse of the cell. The energy mechanisms are dependant on the functions of the mitochondria. Instead the mitochondria in the cells of females are more powerful ! We wondered: did the worshippers of Devi Durga see the dance of female mitochondria !

My *Swabhaav* has generally tended to find the shortest route. I have considered that the shortest distance between two points is a straight line. But a person in search of shortest route can end up cutting corners. This can lead to accidents. I was soon to realize that learning stem cell science through textbooks will also involve similar hazards.

The time honoured route to become a surgeon is to undergo residency training for at least 4 years. My university in Gujarat permitted an alternate route of 5 years that can be pursued after having taught as a tutor in anatomy for 1 year. Utterly naïve, in the very first year of my exposure to clinical medicine as an intern, I wondered how nice it would be to derive some income as a tutor in anatomy and still be a surgeon albeit only a little later. At that time, I was working with a missionary surgeon at Limbdavalu (I.P. Mission) Hospital, Anand. Dr. Rutherford was the Chief without the usual demeanour of surgeons of that time. He would invite interns to his residence, feed us and play harmonium after dinner. So I ventured to ask him about the alternate route.

His reply was, "If you want to learn swimming, you have to jump in the water. Without dirtying your hands, what kind of surgeon would you make?"

I understood, and walked along the well-charted path to be a surgeon.

For the emerging science of stem cell, where are the institutions, the guides and the mentors in India?

We had registered as delegates when we came to know that Indian Science Congress is holding its annual conference at Ahmedabad, Gujarat in 2005. We had great expectations. National conferences dedicated to our disciplines have always discussed recent advances. Indian National Science Congress was indeed a jamboree of science, that the scientists should be celebrating the national and international achievements of the last year. Since independence, the inauguration of the conference was done by the Prime Minister of India. This time one of India's greatest scientist, President A.P.J. Abdul Kalam was also to be there. Some Nobel laureates were also invited.

Glancing through the pages of brochures, I realized that most of the presentations could have been a doctorate thesis. There were no Nobel Laureates. Disappointed, I called home to tell Rajni not to take the trouble, since there does not seem to be anything about stem cells. So I went alone trying to keep an open mind. A notable feature of the Science Congress was the inclusion of every subject that had even the slightest pretence to be science. I attended a few presentations in home science section. It was good to know that we should use all types of cooking oils in a cyclical fashion. Similarly, it was essential to have different types of pulses in the diet to ensure that all 13 essential amino acids were included in the diet. Omega-3, an essential fatty acid, was a new discovery for me. Yet, I had not seen anything about stem cells. I was happy to be proven wrong as seen by narrated happening in an earlier chapter. I was thinking of leaving without attending the last half-day of the conference. But another happening was yet to happen. I saw Dr. Naushir Antia walking towards me. He asked me,

"Bhaskar, what are you doing here?"

"Sir, the father of modern Indian plastic surgery, what are you doing here?"

"I am presenting a paper!" he said.

This was not listed in the brochure ! I sat down for the concluding session as a courtesy to a senior pioneering colleague. Little did I know that it was to pay rich dividends. There were two presentations—one was about the stem cells from limbal region of the eye by Prof. Balu followed by practical applications of cultured limbal stem cells for damaged cornea by Virendra Sangwan, an ophthalmic surgeon. They invited us to L.V. Prasad Eye Institute and later, facilitated a scientist to learn culture expansion of limbal stem cells.

We followed up our quest by attending two more Indian National Science Congresses at Hyderabad and at Chidambaram as narrated earlier.

We wrote a collaborative project with Dr. Shridhar Rao, which was aimed at providing a skin substitute. Burn injuries are widespread in India. As a plastic surgeon, I had looked forward to create such a substitute for a long, long time. Shinya Yamanaka won a Nobel Prize for a research based on a somatic skin cell that can be translated to a pluripotent cell in 2012. We ventured to mention this in our project as a futuristic possibility ! The project did not succeed. A scientist from GoI (Government of India), Shashikumar who was working for SBIRI called up one evening. He said, "The project was brilliantly written. But GoI is interested in finding and funding such projects that will benefit at a large scale the common masses. Your business plan and marketing strategy are really poor."

Shashikumar was a thorough gentleman, he did not expect and I repeat, he did not expect any kickbacks.

Subsequently, when I was next in New Delhi, I met Shashikumar at his residence and learnt from him how to write budgets, marketing strategies and business plans!

After our first successful funding we paid a courtesy call to Shashikumar. This time, on a Sunday morning, he met us on the grounds of a huge school campus. He happened to be the executive trustee of the foundation. He was very happy for us but politely declined to accept a small donation to the school trust. He gracefully accepted a small toy for his recently born son.

Shashikumar had explained his *Swabhaav* thus, we are a generation born after Independence. We have understood the merit for an upright self-respecting personality. We have also understood the need for an outreach beyond bureaucracy. You may call this a personal virtuous trait; we would like it simply to be a further extension of performing our duties.

We would have wished that this personal perception of the duties of a government servant would be widespread. But we understand that generalizations could be erroneous. Shashikumar was bound to rise in hierarchy and may have even retired by now. Suffice it to say that he was truly a good Samaritan.

Shashikumar's suggestion that we pay a courtesy call to Prof. Padmanabhan (he was the chair of the interviewing committee for the projects) proved invaluable.

I had asked:

"Are you sure? No, no. This would amount to approaching the examiner before the exam."

"The times have changed. And, so have the personalities. Even New Delhi is not the same as it was a decade ago. Be sure that Dr. Padmanabhan is astute enough to weed out the chaff from the wheat."

I wrote out a short request with the subject 'Guidance for unsuccessful project'. Prof. Padmanabhan promptly granted an appointment to meet on 26th January!

A post-graduate student ushered me into the office of Prof. Padmanabhan. Yes, there was no mistake. It was 26th January, a national holiday and the professor had already performed the duty to salute the national flag!

He was kind to the extent, a first formal meeting would permit. There was no hectoring nor condescending. Most of the discussions, lasting for about an hour, was about how to write the project. Only assertion that the learned professor made was not to show off what and how much one knows. He explicitly said that mentioning the translation of a somatic cell to pluripotent stem cell by Shinya Yamanaka was not warranted. He concluded by saying that we should write a fresh proposal so that the expert committee would get a just estimation of the scientific merit as well as how the money spent by Government of India would ultimately percolate to a larger benefit of large masses.

The meeting fructified. We were granted two projects in next two years. The first project enabled us to provide scientific proof that mesenchymal stem cells in our laboratory have the potential to translate into the three primary derm layers (ectoderm, that gives rise to neural tissue and skin, mesoderm that gives rise to muscles, bones, connective tissue, and endoderm that gives rise to glandular tissue). We selected diabetes as an application instead of an adjuvant to cancer therapy as we felt that this was best suited for the brief of 'affordable product' for a large population on a long term duration.

Subsequently, we were awarded another project with a bigger amount. Our aim was to make a product that would at least delay if not eliminate the need for joint replacement in osteoarthritis of the knee. It was a herculean task that tested our capabilities to the hilt especially as we had to finish the project in a specified time and money. We will deal with it in a later chapter. It will be appropriate to discuss some scientific aspects concerning stem cells.

9
Open Sesame!

Having begun from zero, we barely began to understand the difference between cell and stem cell. We began by reading the first chapter in *Gray's Anatomy*. *Gray's Anatomy* is an epitome of what the scientific genius of human endeavour can achieve. The book was to be read and learnt in the first year of medical studies. Our curriculum found it unnecessary to study the first chapter that began with the study of a cell. But now reading this chapter was a delightful discovery.

We both were anatomists first and surgeons second. This was a prerequisite to being a good surgeon. We had no knowledge of cell structure and function and hence began a pleasant pursuit.

We refresh that human life begins with a single cell. When an ovum gets fertilized with a spermatozoa—(there are millions of sperms in a single ejaculate of semen and only one is needed to fertilize an ovum)—two of them merge to produce a single cell. This is embryonic pluripotent cell.

Fusion of ovum and spermatozoa occurs within Fallopian tube. A single cellular 'human being to be' continues to float in the Fallopian tube while it continues to subdivide. This further divides and sub-divides without further differentiation into a mass of cells (embryonic stem cells).

The mass would be the size of a very small strawberry, at this point Rajni interrupted:

"A very small strawberry will also be too large. The mass consisting of 8/16/32 or so cells will be a miniscule mass."

"Yes, true. But the image seen by us in the textbook of these few cells reminds me of the image of a strawberry." This mass of cells gets implanted into the inner lining of the uterus—endometrium—how will it stick to the endometrium? Then one of the cells 'decides' to chart out a distinct individualistic course for itself. This is how it will form a distinctly different human being. The result of two of the cells deciding to do this would lead to identical twins. Such siblings are two different human beings with the same genetic structure. If more than one sperm were to fertilize more than one ovum, there can be still twins, triplets and rarely more but they do not have an identical genetic structure. Each of these cells are pluripotent stem cells meaning they are able to grow (i.e., differentiate) into all derivatives that constitute a human body... How the pluripotent stem cells go on to form different organs is explained with a highly philosophical term—morphogenetic fields.

Morphogenetic fields as a concept was a new revelation to us. We had thought that it was a philosophical preset. We had heard about it from Rohit Mehta. Once when he stayed with us after returning from England, we saw that he was fascinated with the term. Every now and then he will quote, Rupert Sheldrake and talk about 'his theory' of morphogenetic fields. Rupert Sheldrake is a theosophist and Rohit Mehta had interacted with him in Theosophical Society, London. Only when we started talking to the scientists in the fields of zoology, did we realize that the concept is scientifically well articulated. Rupert Sheldrake is a hardcore scientist, yet he had speculated about a concept that he called as 'morphic resonance'. We better restrict our discussion only to morphogenetic fields and leave the subject of 'morphic resonance' to the parapsychologists. How morphogenetic fields operate is poorly understood.

We have understood that the universe is governed by 4 fundamental laws of physics. They could also govern a physical organism. Although it is difficult to fathom how they would affect the spatial and temporal side. A *morphogenetic field* is generated by a group of cells or a single stem cell. Cells are able to respond to discrete, localized biochemical signals leading to the development of specific organs. The *spatial* and *temporal* extents of the physical forces are not well understood but beyond simple biochemistry and for sure will be dictated by such physical realities.

We speculated about what is the nature of a morphogenetic field. Surely it cannot be a fundamental weak or strong nuclear force and it cannot be a gravitational force as well. Each and every living system generates an electro-magnetic field. We, therefore, believe that morphogenetic field would be a specific kind of electro-magnetic force that gives special properties to a stem cell. Such an explanation would certainly leave God aside. Let the forces of Nature prevail. The cell biologists are content to accept the belief that there is a morphogenetic field. It guides a group of cells to a distinctly defined spatial location as a cell 'destined' to become part of the liver will go the space where the liver is to be located and formed and so on. Once a stem cell translates to a definitely defined organ, it loses its 'stem-ness'. Therefore, a liver cell may subdivide but it can only regenerate liver. A skin cell may divide, but it can only regenerate skin. Nature has so designed that a pluripotent stem cell must give up its pluripotency once it reaches its destination. But, the regeneration faculty is to be preserved. This is evident in the Mesenchymal stem cell.

Mesenchymal stem cells are present at various locations in the body in different quantities. They are most abundant in fatty tissue under the skin. Another location for their large population is in the bone marrow. It is postulated that this kind of cell responds to the call of Nature whenever there is a need for regeneration. In such a situation they will mobilize themselves to hone to the site of need. We believe that this will not be on a count of any teleologic—(designed by God)—principle but would be most likely because of morphogenetic fields so generated in case of need.

With this understanding, we decided to focus our research onto the study and application of Mesenchymal stem cells. Incidentally it so happened that this was a permissible area of research. Subsequently, there was abundance of researchers all over the planet focusing their attention on this particular stem cell. If there was a question about the existence of a phenomena termed as consilience, here was a proof that it existed.

We spent a modest amount of money from our pension fund

to upgrade our rudimentary stem cell laboratory to a GMP Class-5 laboratory. GMP means Good Manufacturing Practice and cells processed with a view to administer them to human beings should at least have a GMP Class-5 facility. We never believed in setting modest goals and this time was no exception. We decided that we will focus on trying to translate mesenchymal stem cells into all three germinal layers. Prof. Ramesh Bhonde (Professor of Zoology, NCCS, Pune) facilitated with a change in direction. He advised us to focus on adipose derived mesenchymal stem cells instead of bone marrow. That was easy and simple. Our plastic surgeon colleagues in Vadodara were generous to supply lipoaspirates that they were throwing away following cosmetic surgery. We searched for standard protocols for trigerminal translation. In contrast to the practice in medical profession, where we pride in sharing our knowledge and innovations, we have realized that hardcore scientists hold their research protocol close to their chests. If and when they share, they expect a financial return. Prof. Bhonde bucked the tide and was generous enough to give us the protocols available at his laboratory without any expectation of financial gain. This empowered us and in collaboration with Prof. Gopal Kundu we submitted our project to SBIRI. We were successful and the work to cultivate insulin secreting cells for ADMSC started. More on this project later. Subsequently, we came across a fantastic book written by Dr. S. Janarthanan & Dr. S. Vincent. They have published almost all the protocols that a scientist may need for conducting research in biotechnology. Hence, we could translate mesenchymal stem cells from adipose tissue into a nerve cell and a chondrocyte with only a small financial outlay.

We happened to discuss the matter with our erstwhile colleague, Dr. B.S. Anantram. Dr. Anantram, after qualifying as one of India's foremost plastic surgeon, had demurred whether to relinquish his professional career to serve a larger cause, i.e., management of the charitable institutions and hospitals financed by Hegde Trust. He continued to serve mankind by treating patients at Annasawmy Mudaliar General Hospital. Anantram was fascinated by the research and urged us to publish our research as Indian Innovations. Little did we realize that when we said, yes, it would entail a fine chiselling of each and every word before publication in the *Indian Journal of Plastic Surgery*.

Mesenchymal stem cells obtained from bone marrow and adipose tissue are similar in their properties. Both of them have potential to be taken from bench to bedside, a cell such as cardiomyocyte (heart cell that can be seen to pulsate in a petri dish!), obtained by a process in the laboratory will retain only the properties of a heart cell and will lose the property of being a stem cell. A stem cell can be transformed—academically spoken as 'can be translated', into an insulin producing cell. These cells will have similar properties to the insulin producing cells from pancreas. They will respond to glucose stimulation by releasing insulin. They would have lost their stem-ness

Let us see what constitutes 'stem-ness'. The properties of stem cells will differ depending upon the kind of stem cell.... A single embryonic stem cell, produced by the union of a sperm and an ovum (discussion about twins is not relevant here) has the potential to bring about a new human being, with differentiation into specific organs. The embryonic cell will also lose its property with further differentiation into three specific germinal layers. This we have seen before.

Cells that give rise to various components of blood are hematopoietic stem cells. They are present all throughout life in bone marrow. This is widely researched and, is used therapeutically in over 150 conditions.

Pluripotent stem cells are those that have the capacity to generate any of the cell types in the human body. How do the cells forming different organs find their location to form an organ, say liver or heart or kidney, is highly mystical. It is postulated that a particular cell type will have a specific kind of 'field' so that it finds its way to the specific location. This field, called morphogenetic field, is yet to be completely understood since several different disciplines will have to focus together.

In the search for the ultimate, a complete organism, named sheep 'Dolly' was produced by transforming a somatic cell to induced pluripotent stem cell. Such a search at times translates into intense quest and frenzy. To be the first one to come out with an invention has produced some weird situations.

Soon after Shinya Yamanaka was awarded a Nobel Prize, *Nature* published a breakthrough. The article cited research that the authors had been successful in producing a pluripotent stem cell simply by exposing them to a very low *p*H. Scientists from Japan published the research in 2014 and it initially took the scientific world by a storm. What a quantum jump for regenerative medicine! Scepticism of the research quickly rose and as soon as the next issue, in an editorial, *Nature* apologized for printing the research. Subsequently, the research was retracted! This was only in the second time in its history that *Nature* had to apologise for its content.... In 1988, it had published research that water retains memory of substances previously dissolved in it. This had practitioners of homoeopathy awash with delight. As the results could not be replicated, *Nature* had to retract the publication.

A philosopher of research in science, Thomas Kuhn, has concluded that science progresses with falsification of earlier 'established' theories. So shall we keep on making blunders so that scientific research may have a quantum jump?

Our introduction to induced pluripotent stem cells came with a handshake with C.M. Habibullah at a symposium on stem cell research in 2010, New Delhi. I participated in the symposium with several volleys and cascades of questions that extended to even genomics. C.M. Habibullah, who was chairing the session, came across at the conclusion of the session:

"I would like to make a clone of you!"

"Sir, do not, please do not punish with another existence!"

"No, this is a reward for your scientific spirit."

"If that is indeed so, please oblige me with standard operating procedure as to how you obtain induced pluripotent stem cell (iPSC)."

"Do come over to Hyderabad and ask for whatever you want."

Unfortunately, Dr. Habibullah passed away the next month. His son who inherited his research which regenerates liver cells in patients with cirrhosis using stem cells. This novel approach has attracted patients from all over the world. Dr. Habibullah (Jr.) reiterated his father's invitation. If there was indeed a possibility to propagate human existence as a clone, we would have certainly gone to Hyderabad.

I decided to jettison attending national science conferences thereafter. We had found plenty to learn, but not even elementary stem cell research.

Having already accepted Dr. Kundu's invitation to the International conference at Lonavala, we did attend. We understood what translational research exactly meant. So far it had sounded as a high literary metaphor. What the high priests of science were endeavouring was to derive a meaningful, clinical application of their basic research. I also learnt that discovery of a new drug at that time would cost approximately $120 million and journey from bench to bedside application was likely to take about 10-12 years. No wonder none of the high *Pundits* had accomplished this.

Most delegates were from USA with the team leader as Bharat Aggarawal (the now disgraced biochemist from the M.D. Anderson Institute, Texas…! A few presentations on turmeric were presented with clinical evidence. Most of the work was focused on molecular biology. Not a single one on stem cells !

On the positive side, there was the opportunity to develop the scientific relation with Gopal Kundu.

"I am happy that you came. Now you can ask for whatever you want from my laboratory. I expect that my research will progress soon to monkeys!"

"We would like to characterize stem cells from our laboratory with CD markers."

"We will do that. A scientist, Pompom…."

"Why do you call her pompous?"

"No, she is not pompous, her name is Pompom. She will do CD markers for you and train a scientist from your laboratory with the technique."

Most of the scientists left the conference by lunch time. Looking at the beautiful landscape of mountain and hills, with a few fluffy white clouds floating beneath the hills, I found it difficult to move away. Bharat Aggarawal finished some paperwork and when he looked around, we were the only two left in the venue. He asked:

"Oh, you are here! What are you doing?"

"I am musing on the mystical presence. And I am singing a poem in my mind. Listen to what...."

I recited a few lines from the sonnet. It is so pertinent and appropriate to reproduce the poem here:

"What is this life if, full of care,
We have no time to stand and stare.

No time to stand beneath the boughs
And stare as long as sheep or cows.

No time to see, when woods we pass,
Where squirrels hide their nuts in grass.

No time to see, in broad daylight,
Streams full of stars like skies at night.

No time to turn at Beauty's glance,
And watch her feet, how they can dance.

No time to wait till her mouth can
Enrich that smile her eyes began.

A poor life this if, full of care,
We have no time to stand and stare."

Bharat Aggarawal wondered and asked, "What is the relevance here?"

"I think the villagers roundabout are happier than most of us. They have all the time to bask in the glory of Mother Nature. I feel, our relentless pursuit of science is also a different kind of greed. By the way, please tell me what you consider as your best research?"

"Alpha TNF."

I was amazed!

"You discovered Alpha Tumour Necrosis Factor? And you did not submit this towards a Nobel Prize?"

"I did not care."

In the ambience of high intellectualities, I was in a state of innocent naivety. Alpha Tumour Necrosis Factor is a molecule secreted by large cells in blood and similarly in tissues at the time of injury. The discovery has contributed significantly to understanding the process of inflammation. This was a huge step towards understanding the process of inflammation. I was in a state of awe and wondered as to why had this great scientist not been awarded his due ? It turns out that he was stating the truth but not the whole truth! We met Prof. Mande, the newly appointed Director of NCCB. He was meant to be more open-minded in sharing research and less conservative in his approach. Two surprises awaited when Gopal Kundu conducted me to him…. Kundu introduced me as Prof. Vyas, researcher at M.S. University. And Director Mande was even more affable and amicable than what I had heard. He had only one question:

"Why does he not conduct the research at M.S. University?"

"Prof. Bharat Chattoo is doing genomics. They have no facility for marker studies."

I believe Mande was a worshipper of Saraswati. Approached differently with a recommendation from Prime Minister's Office, he had to correspond for about 3 weeks. Thereafter his office quoted an exorbitant quote to train a scientist from our laboratory for 5 days. The figure was just short of 7 digits! Earlier, Lalita Limaye had sat with me for half a day to familiarize me with her laboratory and the work on hematopoietic stem cells !

Soon after, Pompom facilitated a scientist from our laboratory to conduct CD 44 marker study. The result of this study was indicative that the spindle shaped cell cultured in our laboratory was indeed a Mesenchymal stem cell.

We wrote a collaborative project with Gopal Kundu. It was awarded a research grant from Department of Biotechnology, Government of India.

I was with Anant Marathe, team member at TPC at the time. We were ushered in for the presentation. Prof. Padmanabhan welcomed us loudly:

"Here are the researchers from Vadodara. They are being mentored by Prof. Chattoo."

Instinctively we guessed, we seemed to have already won. There were only few questions from experts.

"What is the source of your technology?"
"Technology for isolation of MSC is available as open-access."
"What is your innovation?"
"Translation of MSCs to insulin secreting cells."
"Why do you prefer to investigate Mesenchymal Stem Cells?"
"This cell line is likely to help diabetic and cancer patients."
"What is your preferred choice?"
"Diabetes."
"Why do you prefer this modality?"
"Diabetes is recognized as a national priority."
"Do you have the protocol?"
"Yes, here is a hard copy."

In a short time, we were informed that we had been successful in our application and steps were outlined as to how the funds were to be utilised and what processes were to be followed.... There was a reminder that as collaborator, Gopal Kundu should make himself available when a team for due diligence would be deputed from DBT to Vadodara. As it happened, Gopal Kundu could not be available on the specified date. Prof. Sheshagiri, the chief of the three member team said, "Never mind, are you prepared to go ahead alone?" There was no alternative but to say yes.

10
Frayed Feathers, Ruffled Relationships

It is said that life is relationships. No man is an island. Bridges will have to be built. Friendship is a pure, primordial glue, when there are no barters or kickbacks.

Yet, in spite of there being very few thieves, all houses have latches and locks!

If trust in the innate honesty of human beings and willingness to forgive mistakes made by friends were standard norms of conducting relationships, so much animosity would be avoided.

We begin with a frank admission of utter naivety in ourselves that such ideas would prevail when we established new friendships and collaborations. Stem cell research needed fundamental support from basic scientists, academics from life sciences (from embryologists to immunologists and zoologists). All of them would contribute to concept formation. To provide proof of concept, once again a wide range of clinicians such as pathologists, pharmacologists and specialists in the field of clinical medicine would need to collate. Cooperative collaborations are rising globally. However, two primary areas of interest, we are now learning to understand, will persist: Pecuniary rewards for the work performed and even more importantly need for respect and status. High priests in academics, once in a while retorted: It is elementary, no payment, no work done. We had to muse silently in our mind that we thought this was the prime motive of the proletariat. Rare are the people of the class of Prof. Ramesh Bhonde. He was one of the rare few who did not count money as a reward and rather took pride in getting some of his conceptual ideas being published as clinical research.

Prof. Ramesh Bhonde is one of the foremost researchers on stem cells nationally. He was the person who kindled the interest for stem cell research at M.S. University, Vadodara. Prof. Bhonde conducted his research in an environment replete with sophisticated equipment. Flow cytometric studies and confocal microscopic images were prerequisites for publishing his research in international journals. However, he had his feet soundly grounded on Earth. He firmly believed that for a clinician wanting to apply his concepts to patients need not indulge in such superlative luxuries…

We heard Prof. Ramesh Bhonde delivered a lecture at the M.S University for the first time. His elegant presentation described how to translate a mesenchymal stem cell into insulin producing cell and later on progress to produce a virtual islet cell aggregate took our fancy to unfathomable heights! What a wonder! What a miracle! In the intermission, Prof. Bhonde, contrary to our expectations was candidly a simple person. He instantaneously said yes to our request for help. When asked for the remuneration, he simply said, "We will see." And he has been true to his spoken word ever since.

His view of the regulations and approvals was also perfunctory. A research should be honestly well conceived. Proof of concept should be derived with well conducted clinical studies. Animal experiments are an unnecessary sacrifice: They are necessary only at the fundamental science level. Animal studies need not include a whole gamut of animals: a few mammalian experiments conducted at well reputed laboratories should suffice as evidence. With the primary motivation to help a fellow human being who may not have an alternative source for redressal, stem cell therapy may be offered with mutual informed consent. That would involve the recipient/ family of the patient and the team of the researcher.

It was this generous understanding of the ground situation in clinical medicine by Prof. Bhonde that we formulated two projects (pertaining to Diabetes Mellitus and Osteoarthritis) that were funded by the Department of Biotechnology, Government of India. Dr. Damodar Nene, a second generation Maharashtrian living in Vadodara is a thoroughbred literary writer. Maharashtra incarnate himself. Under his presidentship we felicitated Prof. Ramesh Bhonde as *Maharashtra Ratna* at Vadodara.

More on this in another chapter. At this juncture, there is a cross-current with our research applications and hypnosis. We invited Prof. Nagaraja, Director of National Institute of Mental Health and Allied Sciences (NIMHANS) to attend a conference on Hypnosis at Vadodara. He was a man of few words and high simplicity.... In one of the sessions, he sat near me and in between the presentation discussed what is yet unknown about this altered state of consciousness. While wishing him a farewell, we asked, "Shall we research genomics of the hypnotic state?" When he answered with a simple yes, little did we realize that he was making a huge commitment.

Some time later, he wrote to us that he had discussed the matter with the Secretary of the Department of Biotechnology. There was a possibility that the project on genomics and molecular biology of hypnosis could be written. The project cost was around Rs. 6 crore for a period of 3 years. Obviously, we were delighted at this prospect. We demurred about a possible diversion from stem cell research to brain physiology.

We received a proposal which was written by Prof. Nagaraja as principal investigator and five high profile scientists from the Indian Institute of Science, Bangalore. We were to be collaborators. We returned the signed copies to Prof. Nagaraja when he visited Gandhinagar soon after.

Our excitement knew no bounds. Little did we realise what lay ahead.

We spoke to Prof. Nagaraja about our research association with Prof. Chattoo and that he was closely associated with the network for funding at Department of Biotechnology. Prof. Chattoo had expressed a desire to be associated with this research.

We asked Prof. Nagaraja:

"Would it be possible for Prof. Chattoo to be involved with the project?"

"No, not at all. I have known him as an expert in plant genomics."

"Prof. Chattoo has a well equipped genomics laboratory. That includes even micro array facilities. Dose NIMHANS have this facility?"

"We will acquire it when funding will be granted. It will be a part of the proposal."

The conversation between two high profile researchers did not go smoothly. Prof. Chattoo was unlike any Kashmiri Pandit we had met. He wanted to be a partner in making a contribution to human genomics. Ground breaking research on the altered states of consciousness was to be conducted for the first time. Gene expressions showing differential protein synthesis responsible for the euphoric state after hypnosis would be detected. This would expand our understanding about the regenerative effects seen after hypnosis.

On the other hand, Dr. Nagaraja got impatient. He said, "All this is understood and well written in our proposal. We will consider your participation at a later date!" And he cut off the phone abruptly.

Prof. Chattoo was a hugely respected academic. On entering packed auditoriums, sight of the erudite professor evoked an awed silence. Such an abrupt ending of a conversation would have been humiliating. We apologised to him and he was gracious to wave it away. He said, "I wish I had been able to make a humble contribution."

Our understanding is that such insults cause immense hurt and are difficult to reconcile. Human tendency is to look for revenge. We know that human history would be different if the instinctual impulse for retaliation was to be sublimated by forgiving and forgetting the insult.

Rajni has always shown generosity to family and friends by her ability to forgive. On the other hand, I have often been brash and hurtful in my behaviour. It is now that I appreciate that my friends and family have been kind to me at these times.

Tide was about to turn.

Little did Prof. Nagaraja think that NIMHANS would find a director to replace him. He repeatedly spoke about the TINA factor. "There is no alternative to Nagaraja!" Although he continued to be a professor at NIMHANS, he was no longer its director. We were disappointed but hardly surprised. The only constant factor in worldly affairs is change. For the presentation at the Department of Biotechnology, New Delhi; Prof Nagaraja deputed a colleague. I was the second member selected to appear before the panel.

Dr. Habibullah who was chairing read out the comments from two experts.

One of the experts had made a detailed analysis of the abilities of each of the six principal investigators for six sub-sections. He had extensively researched the relevant publications on the subject. His conclusion was that this research may contribute to further understanding of genomics of consciousness at a human level, including the altered state of consciousness. Final comment: Recommended.

Second expert had a single line comment: Funding this research will be a huge wastage of public resources!

The project was rejected.

At the end of the session, Prof. Habibullah indicated that he wished to chat. As I went near him in a loud voice that was intended to be heard by all, he said "Department of Biotechnology wants to establish a few centres of excellence across the country. M.S. University, Vadodara, is teaching in English medium. Research capability at your university is well recognized. Would you like to take this message to the Vice Chancellor, so that the University may apply to be a centre of excellence?"

We promptly carried out his wishes and took his message to Prof. Ramesh Goyal, the then Vice Chancellor of M.S. University. He was quick to respond. We had no hesitation in recommending a department who had been actively collaborating with us. The said department won a grant for Rs. 13.5 crore and was nominated a centre for excellence.

Although the research was on an even keel, we needed a quantum jump. We were hopeful that this would bring further collaboration and progress in the research. Alas it was not to be! Our request to be recognised as a centre for Ph.D. study was turned down. We slowly saw a decrease in the amount of collaboration and eventually our emails remained unanswered.

11
Turnabout and Turncoat Idealism

Ramesh Bhonde advised a change of direction after we have studied the bone marrow derived mesenchymal stem cells for a few years. Bone marrow should be replaced by adipose tissue. We preferred this option as well. (I have performed plenty of lipo suction procedures as a plastic surgeon). Adipose tissue is easier to obtain and abundant in quantity. Bone marrow would yield about 10 per cent MSCs; while lipoaspirate will yield 30-40 per cent. Dr. Anant Marathe had joined us. When we submitted the research project to DBT, Prof. Bhonde readily offered to be a mentor.

Prof. Bharat Chattoo was so far advising us about genomics. We could not afford to conduct micro array assays in human genomics as it was prohibitively expensive. We found an article in *Nature* that could potentially provide a short cut and reduce the costs. We set up a meeting with Prof. Chattoo.

However, the professor curtailed the meeting. "Yes, it is feasible. There is yet another short cut available. You can study a limited number of genes that modulate consciousness. Thereafter whatever proteins that such genes encompass, either by their expression or suppression can be further studied in a dry laboratory. This is a new tool laboratory—bioinformatics."

We have discussed this with Ernest Rossi. Rossi had an elegant logistic hypothesis. He had postulated that a hypnosis therapy session conducted in the altered state of consciousness, with certain manipulations in syntax will change the semantics. This message will pass on to the genes (!) From immediate early onset certain genes will be expressed or indeed maybe suppressed. We had published a paper related to this in a *American Journal of Clinical Hypnosis*. We thought Prof. Chattoo would like to discuss this further.

When I tried to elaborate Prof. Chattoo cut me short. He asked,

"I understand you have applied for a DBT grant."
"Yes, but it is about stem cell research."
"Do you know that I am a member of the expert committee?"
"Yes, but we thought to discuss it would be imprudent."

He rang up a mobile number. He asked, "When are you likely to schedule the visit by the experts to TPC, Vadodara?"

Thus, we came to know that we seemed to have succeeded. Secondly, we understood that Prof. Bharat Chattoo was in a commanding situation.

Soon, we received a communication from Small Business Innovation Research Initiative—SBIRI. A team of 3 members were to visit us for due diligence. We were surprised to note that we are not required to arrange for their reception at the airport. Transport was being organised by their department. We were not required to provide lunch either. Only a cup of tea and biscuits were permitted!

We were pleasantly surprised to see this new face of India that we had envisaged in our dreams. It truly reflected the personality of the head of the visiting team.

Prof. Sheshagiri was in a strict vigilance mode. One by one he verified that we had the equipment that we had shown in the documents to be in our possession. He saw mesenchymal stem cells in our laboratory. He verified that CD 44 marker studies were conducted at NCCS, Pune. At this point he double checked, is it sure that Prof. Gopal Kundu cannot make it to Baroda today, and moved on quickly to review few proofs of concept studies that we had conducted. When he was busy reading our publications, the other two experts were more than satisfied. Without realizing that I was standing at a hearing distance, they spoke to each other, "Some researchers have taken more than 1 crore. And have not done even half of what these people have already done." At this stage we disclosed to the non-scientific, financial expert that we have changed the name of the company from Total Potential Cell Pvt. Ltd. to Total Potential Cells Pvt. Ltd. We tried to explain that this was necessary because we had to withdraw from the Biotech Park, Savli. After 3 years of waiting, there was no development of the incubator that had been promised by Gujarat State Biotechnology Mission—GSBT. The incubator space was well cordoned off and yet, in spite of any building with sophisticated equipment, one can see only donkeys grazing around there.

He was not interested. He said, "All the same, TPC remains TPC. Correct?" We replied, "Yes. Same promoters, same researchers and same team. Only a new names."

The execution and successful completion of the project happened to be a hefty challenge. Procuring 20 samples of lipoaspirates was easy. Our practicing plastic surgery friends were generous to supply large quantities of lipoaspirates. The rest of the process was an arduous task. We had to decide whether to do enzymatic digestion with trypsin or a chemical processing with a toxic substance, Fecol. We had to wait to make sure that we obtained pure mesenchymal stem cells. We managed to procure MSCs with more than 90 per cent purity after passaging twice!

The study of cell markers on mesenchymal stem cells is an expensive task. Even the supplier of the cell markers, needed to be carefully assessed about their capabilities. Regardless, the cell markers are expensive. We wasted an entire batch of positive and negative cell markers. No refunds! We found a guardian angel, Dr. Ansarullah who happened to be on sabbatical leave in Vadodara at this time. He selected a second supplier and there was success in store. Dr. Ansarullah, a gentle, self-effacing professorial person had spent a few years in United States in Stanford University. His post-doctoral research was also on the same topic: 'Translation of mesenchymal stem cells to produce insulin cell aggregates.'

Dr. Ansarullah who preferred to be called as Ansar Aman (Aman translates from Urdu to English as peace) gave a lot of peace. He not only found the right supplier for the dye studies, helped in the characterization with four positive stem cell markers but also helped in establishing a protocol for translation of mesenchymal stem cells to insulin producing cells. He took the ICAs from our laboratory to conduct confocal microscope studies at Prof. Chattoo's laboratory. When we reviewed the confocal microscope pictures, we saw the peak of Mt. Everest right before our eyes!

Dr. Ansar stayed at Vadodara for about a year. He wanted to stay in India if a suitable research facility and salary that he well deserved—Rs. 6 lakh per annum—were to be available. Mother India could not nurture this worthy erudite professor. He is now working in Germany so that the entire planet may benefit. His stay in Vadodara was instrumental to our success.

In addition Dr. Ansar mentored Jaymesh Thadani, our senior most scientist. Together they perfected the protocols for isolation, culture and expansion of mesenchymal stem cells to islet aggregates. They also produced 500 islet cell like aggregates that secreted insulin. They conducted the tests to prove ICAs did secrete insulin in the laboratory. That paved the way for implantation of ICAs in the liver in 6 patients with diabetes.

The year pleasantly went by in the pursuit of what was thought to be an impossible task. The task was achieved through the efforts and ingeniousness of several members of the team.

We presented the research at the annual function of BIRAC 2015, with Rajni as the presenter. We won the best research award for 2015. Even then we hardly realized that we have established a significant milestone for finding a resolution to several problems faced by patients with diabetes.

Prof. Bharat Chattoo was even more pleased than us. He egged us on to think about yet another research application. Department of Biotechnology had formulated a Business Ignition Grant (BIG). BIG aimed at funding such research proposals that can be taken up for a lasting business adventure. We were advised to continue with further application in the diabetic domain. Wisdom would lie in repeating what we have already done before. But that would not be suitable to our psychological profile. We decided to apply for a grant to see if we could achieve mesenchymal cell translation to chondrocytes. We discovered that such translation studies were successful in animals. But there was no study to show if this had been achieved in humans.

Dr. Anant Marathe and I presented before the expert committee.

The committee burst out into laughter when I replied to the last question that, "Several studies in different animal species have been conducted. That includes bovine, porcine, equine etc. Only elephantine and human species are yet to be studied!"

We understood that we have been successful in being awarded the grant.

It required a lot of effort and a few visits to BIRAC that the previously funded TPC and the current TPC under consideration for funding for a new project are the same people. There is no camouflage; no subterfuge but only a force of circumstance that the incubator at Biotech Park, Savli did not materialize. Finally, when BIRAC was convinced that the same researchers, same promoters are using the funding, that they released the funds after much delay.

We had 6 months to organize the team. We had to find a suitable multi-speciality hospital with more than 80 beds. We had to acquire the added equipment before the start of the project, take ethics committee and stem cell research committee approvals, and so on.

We advertised the commencement of the project in local newspapers. One hundred and thirty eight patients turned up as volunteers! Dr. Pradeep Mehta and Dr. Umang Gandhi had a difficult time in choosing the participants.

There was an opinion that we select only those with Grade 2 osteoarthritis of the knee. That would have given a surely successful result. But that would have diminished the merit of the study. In the end we decided to include in the study those patients, who had both the knees affected with osteoarthritis. We also decided to include Grade 3 and 4 stage of osteoarthritis. The patients with injuries to the cartilages within the knee as well as the ligaments were also included.

We enlarged the number of the knees studied to 50 by including both the knees in 25 patients. All the patients reported satisfactory progress, subjectively and with objective parameters of clinical assessment. We had expected that a new cartilage formation will be evident at the end of one year. There was a disappointment looming large in our minds. None of the MRI studies showed a shadow of a new cartilage formation. Have we failed? Have we failed? Have we failed?

Hope lied in the fact that except one patient, all the others were satisfied and happy. Their pain had gone. Their mobility had increased and other clinical parameters of assessment also showed improvement. With extensive literature search we understood that the type of the regenerated cartilage would be embryonic like cartilage. Moreover it will be very thin. This will be unlikely to show even with MRI. We presented the results to BIRAC. They were satisfied. When presented at Indian Association of Rheumatologist and Orthopaedic Surgeons Conference, the project was awarded Gold medal for the best research.

We were a bit surprised when 2 electronic media, published from Chicago, approached us for a briefing! We had been accustomed to the times when news took a long time to travel through word of mouth. S. Ramesh of *India Post* interviewed on Skype. Laxmanrao of *Chicago Tribune* came personally to Vadodara. *Tamanna* (a periodical) gave coverage twice. Following week, Anant Marathe phoned and we could see that he was bursting with joy. One of his friends had called up from USA and asked, "Anant, we knew that you were carved out to be a big sportsman. But never did we know that you are to make that giant size of a researcher as to climb to Chicago as well!"

Regional Gujarati newspapers and national newspapers including *Times of India* publicized our research. Some researchers, while on their vacation travels to India, came to visit us. They were surprised to have a look at our modest laboratory. They did not doubt the veracity, but advised us to have more sophistication with a view to sell the research.

We started to get a trickle of small number of patients from USA and UK. Apart from monetary help to sustain our research, it provided a big ego booster.

Cerebral Palsy is a disorder that affects newborn and young infants. We have understood that the primary cause of this disorder is insufficient oxygenation to the brain. It was surmised that treatment with mesenchymal stem cells, while the brain is developing, may be beneficial to the children.

A young lady of 30 years, diagnosed with cerebral palsy since many years approached us with her parents. We were persuaded to treat her regardless that the outcome may not be of much avail. This young lady improved so very much that she travelled all across Gujarat, to persuade patients with cerebral palsy to come forward for treatment. Little did she understand that her treatment could be carried out because of their explicit understanding and expressed request. It would require a large scale clinical trial before it could be offered as a treatment on a large scale. When we were flooded with the requests from expectant parents, we decided to conduct a proof of the concept study with 10 patients. Doctor Prof. Usha Modi has been a long time friend. She was a puritan Gandhian: Professionally as well as personally. We had long discussions with her over a few sessions to assure her that there is a possibility that success, even in a limited degree would mean improving the quality of life of these children for the rest of their lives. She was aware of studies from national and international institutes that results were not favourable. She reluctantly agreed to participate on the explicit understanding that the Helsinki protocol will be followed in word and spirit.

We treated 10 patients. 6 out of them improved with the parameters of the milestones that were defined by Prof. Modi. Most remarkable improvement that is sustained today after almost 8 years is of a young girl. She was blind and had to be cared in a cradle till she was 12 years old. She required to be sedated during the transport from Ahmedabad to Vadodara. She was transported in a trunk of the van. Within a year of treatment, she was on her feet. She started going to a blind school and is now undergoing vocational training as a blind person. We hoped to improve her further with some restoration of sight. Her father who had suffered terribly whilst caring for her (he had lost his job as his caring duties took priority) however refused consent for any further treatment. He wanted to rest on her limited gains.

Thus, we were riding high. We prepared a project for stage 1 clinical trial and submitted to Department of Science this time. There were many collaterals including the assessment of cognitive and other functions by child psychologists from Department of Home Science at the University. Over a period of 3 years, the project was estimated to cost Rs. 1 crore.

Along with Rajni, Dr. Anant Marathe, this time Nirupa also went as a presenter. The expert panel consisted of only 3 members. To our pleasant surprise, we found Prof. Ganguly as chairman. In his inimitable style, Dr. Ganguly straightaway focused on Nirupa, "We have heard your mother speak before. We have thought about collaboration with her. I know the academics. I believe that this trial will cost much more than the stipulated budget. Tell me, how are you going to finance the deficit?"

"We will bear the burden as needed." said Nirupa.

"So do you expect your parents to leave you with some debt? I would not like that."

"My expertise is as a finance manager. I will find the money."

"But debts have to be paid. I don't like it." After a pause, Prof. Ganguly said, "Your proposal is rejected. Apply again when you have found some more money. Hopefully that time there will be some other person as chairman."

Rajni interjected at this point, "Yes sir. Everything else may have changed then. There will be one constant factor that Prof. Ganguly will be the chairman!" Everybody burst into laughter including the other 2 experts who were in a silent mode all the time. Although we left laughing, but our enthusiasm to present projects was fast fading.

At this juncture, a lot of advice and some pressure to sell our research started coming. BIRAC, Biotechnology Consortium of India Ltd. (BCIL), C-CAMP advised to hold our hand by mentoring. Research recognition by DSIR was due for renewal. They also asked: "You have been granted customs exemptions for importing your equipment, you would have derived benefit and the government would have lost some revenue. How much is the amount?"

"We have not availed of this benefit at all."

"Even then it is expected that the country should benefit with your research. Your work has been sponsored with public money."

Multinationals from Japan and other countries are buying biotech research from India because valuations appear to be cheap by their standards etc.

So after much persuasion, at the third time, we applied for a Launching Entrepreneurial Affordable Products (LEAP) Project funding. This involved only bare academic details, the emphasis was how the proposal would be attractive to a promising entrepreneur to invest in the equity of a start-up company.

From being academics to now becoming vendors of our research, we were helped by Deepak Raja and Sandeep David. Firstly, we were made to apply for a patent. This was contrary to our ideology. We thought. C.N. Rao produced 400+ products and is still researching for more and did not seek a patent for a single product. We were made to realize that this route was for fierce idealists of the last century who were on a full time salary at a grandiose institution. The idealism may be termed as fantastic idealism since such a fantasy can accrue only a fortunate few. Their entire research funding would have been at public expense. A small entrepreneur with an expensive hobby of biotechnology research will have to generate his own additional resources, even if some public funding was to be available.

We had known that a stem cell is a biological product, a gift of nature. It cannot be patented as per the law. When we began research, we had taken this fact in our stride. We had thought we do not want to go patenting. Let Mother India benefit. We may be called turncoat idealists instead now. We must agree that there is nothing absolute about our idealism. When survival is at stake, even God will forgive us, may even exhort us to be a turncoat. This reminds us of a brilliant lawyer, who had to execute a turnabout; still in service of his client.

The story goes that a lawyer with brilliant eloquence vehemently argued and was about to conclude when his assistant pulled his jacket and passed a short note. "Sir, you have argued in favour of our opponent." Taking a short pause, the lawyer became a turncoat. He continued, "What I said before would be what my learned opponent would say. Now I will quash each argument piece by piece and turn them to figments."

Now we take the solace, if we were to find a buyer for our research, maybe from abroad, Mother India and people at large globally will benefit. Patents have been applied and are in process. We wrote this on the day when India was celebrating *Shankaracharya Jayanti* (28th April). Now Shankara's philosophy is the ultimate as considered by his followers. The axiomatic truth propounded by

Shankaracharya provides the generic ground of a yardstick to measure the veracity of Truth. They are as follows:

1. **prajñānam brahma**—"Prajñāna is Brahman", or "Brahman is Prajñāna"
2. **ayam ātmā brahma**—"This Self (Atman) is Brahman"
3. **tat tvam asi**—"Thou art that"
4. **aham brahmāsmi**—"I am Brahman", or "I am Divine"

All philosophy generated from above into different fields of discipline is relative to not only at the time and at the place but also on who is doing it, why is he doing it, how is he done and with what motivation.

We have defended our actions enough. Call it a survival strategy or term it as turncoat idealism; what matters at the bottom line is survival.

12
At Prime Minister's Office and Thereafter

Project SVISCRTH

We requested an audience with the Dalai Lama to seek his spiritual guidance in our quest to fathom the further depths of consciousness. We had learnt from the book by Howard Benson, '*The Relaxation Response*' that the office of Dalai Lama took about 6 months to answer the letters. We had better luck. Tenzin Geychi, the aristocratic private secretary then, answered with a telegram that we had been granted an audience on 6 September, 1987! Good fortune that it was, we also had an appointment granted by Swami Chinmayanand.

We confirmed with Tenzin Geychi. We requested the manager at Sitbari Ashram to schedule our audience with Swamiji around the same day. Sitbari Ashram telegraphically answered: Do not come. Ashram is full. No vacancy.

With this backdrop, Rajni stayed back. Regardless, I went. Was provided a room at Sitbari Ashram and could meet both! Is it not true that heaven helps those who help themselves? This miracle like situation happened with a connection that was established by Rajni. One of the trustees of the Ashram had his daughter married at Vadodara and Rajni had been her obstetrician! Subsequently, we had several audiences with the Dalai Lama. We published his biography and for the first time in Gujarat, he came to Vadodara, to inaugurate a charitable hospital. We had founded this hospital, along with like-minded friends. Aruna Mehta, more humanist than any radical humanist, who drove herself to frenzy in her attempts like an ant running to donate blood for an injured elephant, led as a President. It began by initially raising small donations by contribution from school children. They had let go of a candy stick or ice cream and donated the money to the trust. The Dalai Lama's visit served as generous blessings to the hospital that is now a multi-crore charitable hospital.

The Dalai Lama visited Gujarat several times thereafter. When he was visiting Vadodara once again, we were pleasantly surprised that the Chief Minister, Mr. Narendra Modi was bracketed with him for more than an hour. This meeting paved the way for holding an international conference on Buddhist heritage at the M.S. University.

At the International Conference, historians from the University presented papers on Buddhist relics in Gujarat. There were several papers from all-over India about Buddhist pilgrimage sites beginning with Sarnath to several other places where Buddhist shrines were located. Picking on this thread, the Chief Minister, Mr. Narendra Modi announced that the Government of Gujarat would initiate a Buddhist trail all-over India so as to attract the Buddhists on a pilgrimage from around the world.

The following week we sent to the Chief Minister, a copy of our biography of the Dalai Lama, 'Experiments with Truth and Non-Violence: China Challenged'. Shri Narendrabhai Modi, acknowledged with a beautiful 'Thank you' card. We thought that to be the completion of a loop.

After some time, we received a letter from the Chief Secretary to the Government of Gujarat, A.K. Sharma. He had asked us for a meeting at Gandhinagar to discuss the Buddhist trail with a suggestion that the Chief Minister might wish us to hold this flag!

We remained in silent contemplation for some time before replying. Our way of life has been so far that of outward participation and inward reconciliation. With ease, we have been happy to include both. Embarking on a historical expedition on a Buddhist trail all over India would mean to live the life like nomads. And how long does an expedition sponsored with political patronage last?

We decided to jettison the idea of a Buddhist trail, but

inspiration came from the Buddhist trail as charted by Samdhong Rinpoche. He is a profound Buddhist scholar, revered as 'Guruji'. He was the Vice Chancellor to Sarnath University. He was the last elected Kalon Tripa—Prime Minister for the Government in exile for Tibet. His final destination has been at McLeodganj, Dharamshala.

We politely declined the visit to Gandhinagar. The Mayor of Vadodara was to accompany and he simply did not understand. We had given an excuse that our research in stem cells was going on and could not be left in mid-way.

In 2014, there was a change of government at New Delhi. Jawaharlal Nehru, as the first Prime Minister of India, had the vision to advance India scientifically to modernity. Subsequent prime ministers had provided token support by inaugurating the National Science Congress year after year. Mr. Narendra Modi sprang a surprise for scientists in India when he decided on his first foreign tour to visit Japan. And at Japan, he visited the laboratory of Prof. Shinya Yamanaka! He saw stem cells of different categories under the microscope. At the conclusion of the Japan visit, he signed a collaboration to advance stem cell research in India.

We insert our letter to the PM:

"Dear Shri Narendra Bhai;
Our Most Respected Prime Minister,
Namaskar!

We acknowledge with deep gratitude an unprecedented debt from Indian scientists, particularly from Gujarat, for your penchant and passion for the furtherance of stem cell research. We wrote to you soon after your return from Kyoto about our successful research to develop Multipotent multilineage stem cells. We had a prompt response from PMO *via* ICMR asking to submit a Project! We are given to understand that the evaluation report on the project will soon be with Mr. Selvakumar at your office."

We knew about Mr. Narendra Modi's fascination for biotechnology and stem cells. We were aware that he had allocated Rs. 60 crore to set up a stem cell facility at Surat, Gujarat. It will be a sad story to dwell upon as to what happened to the proposed and already initiated facility after Mr. Narendra Modi left Gujarat. But we were encouraged by the Japan visit and wrote to him a congratulatory response. The letter apprised him that some of the cells that he saw at Japan were also the topic of research at our modest laboratory. We also mentioned that we had signed MoU with the Government of Gujarat that envisaged setting up a stem cell research laboratory, in addition to facilitation to advance holistic health under the title Swami Vivekananda Institute of Stem Cell Research & Therapy and Holistic Health.

We had a prompt response from the PMO. The dialogue between two secretaries and us went on to 3 meetings and correspondence for several weeks. We would like all the government officials to be role models emulating these gentlemen. They were discrete, polite, highly sensible, and probing with well directing direction. Such a description may as well be liked by most; but we sense that these high profile officials would not like to be mentioned with their proper names. Therefore, we simply mention the first one whom we met as Mr. S.

Mr. S asked for a project report that they intended to be sent to ICMR for evaluation.

We shared the letter with Prof. Chattoo and other friends. Bharat Chattoo shared a few stories similar to the situation. When Mr. Narendra Modi was the Chief Minister, he was asked to prepare projects on genomics and how he regretted that he had given the situation a pass. He was sure that this time we would prepare a detailed project, regardless of the time and enormity of the effort.

The situation sent us into a dizzy. There was a whirlwind of brainstorming. Our scientists rummaged through all the records to weed out chaff from the wheat. In a short time we compiled the material that ran into 200 pages! We abbreviated most of the material with addition of photographs of stem cells from our laboratory to about 30 pages. Of course, there was one photograph of Mr. Narendra Modi too. We sent it to the PMO. The gist of the project SVISCRTAH runs as under:

SWAMI VIVEKANANDA INSTITUTE OF STEM CELL RESEARCH & THERAPY AND HOLISTIC HEALTH (SVISCRTAH)

Project Report

It is proposed to set up Swami Vivekananda Institute of Stem Cell Research & Therapy and Holistic Health in a village near Baroda, Gujarat. The project is inspired by the visit of the Prime Minister Shri Narendra Bhai Modi to Prof. Shinya Yamanaka at Kyoto as well as his successful call at the United Nations General Assembly to celebrate June 21st as the International Yoga Day.

Preamble

The Concept

At the first site, it may appear that Stem Cell Science and Yoga are a disjointed cliché. It will be made clear that both the disciplines are to be approached through the modern scientific discipline.

There are phases in drug discovery. Ayurveda and several modern medicines rely on herbal preparations. Chemical drug discoveries begin with a molecule with surveillance as to the structure of the molecule and though the peak is already passed, a few drugs still go through organic chemistry route with some alterations in the molecular structure. Biologically derived drugs like antibiotics, also have seen the zenith of the achievements and, with the synthesis of Insulin in the laboratory through the Recombinant RNA route has seen a climax whereby active molecules are synthesized in the laboratory.

Twenty-first Century belongs to the next generation of therapeutic innovations which will be derived from cell based therapy and stem cells. Stem cells are the basis for Regenerative and Rejuvenative process in the body from childhood to old age. The myths and unfounded fears that the science based on stem cells may threaten through the development of teratomas and clones have been practically sorted out. The modern science, as well as

ICMR in India has already identified the safe line of cells and stem cells that can be safely researched as well as applied to therapeutics. The Regulatory system, thus treat it in the range of doable category. Several Hematopoietic stem cells are universally in a therapeutic range. It falls upon the Indian geniuses to bring this category of therapeutic stem cell line into affordable healthcare.

Simultaneously, the research and its application in permissible areas of stem cell lines opens up a vast opportunity to get into such other diseases domains like neuro degenerative diseases, Diabetes etc. where India can take the lead and achieve advanced breakthroughs. What China has done in last 10 years, we need to catch up with.

Introduction

More than a decade ago, that time as the Chief Minister of Gujarat, Shri Narendrabhai Modi foresaw Bharat of today equipped with Biotechnology. Gujarat saw the emergence of Gujarat Biotechnology Mission and 2 Biotechnology parks. The leap came about through a quantum jump of budget of Rupees Ten Thousand crore in the Union Budget in 2014-15. There was a visible clear signal when the Prime Minister of India, probably, the first, visited the Nobel laureate Scientist Shinya Yamanaka at Kyoto. It was surely to show which direction the Prime Minister wanted India to move ahead in coming years. It was in the direction of science with a focus on Biotechnology which would make new research to become affordable healthcare for vast masses. Kyoto thus became a symbol of aspiration. The Nobel laureate almost performed a miracle by translating adult somatic cells to Induced Pluripotent Stem Cells—iPS. While, this will be a mother of enunciation to come, as of today iPS, though it is the highest achievement in stem cell science, remains far from clinical application. Before iPS is further researched, that the regulatory bodies clear it for an application in research in Human Domain, there are still several cell lines available within the permissible areas of doable research that have been given the new thrust by the Government of India. The Biotechnology sector is capable now of rapid thrust into establishing the facilities for the therapeutic application of established cell lines and simultaneously utilizing the permissible research cell lines so as to develop a new therapeutic range of stem cell derived medication for so far untreatable medical conditions.

There was another thrust by Shri Narendrabhai Modi as a Prime Minister of India. He sponsored and got it passed at the UN General Assembly that from 2015 the world would celebrate 21st June as the International Yoga Day. It was the Dream of Maharishi Aurobindo that India should emerge as a world teacher. This spiritual aspiration is coming through a pooled circle, now in a scientific paradigm. Last few decades of Advancements in Neuroscience and Psychology have seen the emergence of mind-body-continuum. Numerous Cytokines including Endorphins are established as a product of thought processes. The brain has justifiably established itself as the largest Endocrine gland. The linkages of good and bad thought processes to the particular locations in brain are precisely mapped out. What was esoteric, mystic Rajyoga has been studied through the scientific parameters. Several researchers studied Buddhist meditators (and Buddhist meditation is an elaborate version of various strategic programmes, initiated by Patanjali) who have discovered the healing properties of strategic meditation programmes. What was initially conceptualized as *Yoga Nidra* by Swami Satyananda Saraswati at Bihar School of Yoga, has now been translated under the modern versions of Hypnotherapy all across the Western world. The Bihar School of Yoga was founded in 1964 by Sri Swami Satyananda Saraswati to impart yogic training to householders and *sannyasins* alike. The Yoga techniques developed there are a synthesis of many approaches to personal development, based on traditional Vedantic, tantric and yogic teachings in conjunction with contemporary physical and mental health sciences. Today, these techniques are taught by Bihar Yoga Bharati and also by Satyananda Yoga Academies in Australia and Colombia. At Simonton Health Centre for Breast Cancer, Dr. O. Carl Simonton, a radiation oncologist popularized the mind-body connection in fighting cancer. Early in his medical career, he noticed that patients given the same dose of radiation for similar cancers had different outcomes. When he looked into why, he concluded that people who had a more positive attitude generally lived longer and had fewer side effects. In a study by Stanford University and the University of California, Berkeley researchers concluded in 1989 that women with advanced breast cancer who received emotional counselling lived about twice as long as those who did not. The study was independent evidence that Dr. Simonton's "whole body" approach to battling the illness made a difference. Dr. Atkins Health Centre for Coronary Artery Diseases is one of the few shining examples in the USA. On the other hand, Dr. Nagendra and Dr. Nagratna at Swami Vivekananda Yoga Anusandhana Samsthana at Bangalore are a functioning Holistic Health Model. The Swami Vivekananda Yoga Research Foundation was recognized as a Scientific & Industrial Research Organization (SIRO) from the Department of Scientific & Industrial Research, Ministry of Science & Technology, Government of India in the year 1988 as it started following the path breaking work in evaluating the therapeutic use of yoga in the management of bronchial asthma and in other aspects from 1984. The scientific accomplishments thereafter and the disciplined education based on the science and philosophy of yoga resulted in receiving University affiliations leading to a doctoral level programme in yoga and allied sciences under the Faculty of Science, Bangalore University. Dean Ornish, M.D., is the founder and president of the non-profit Preventive Medicine Research Institute (PMRI). He brings the future of medicine today–the tools to customize a way of eating, managing stress, and exercising that is based on your own desires, needs, and genetic predispositions. **Your genes are not your fate.** New research by the Dean, Dr. Ornish and his colleagues shows that changing what you eat and how you live may actually alter, for the better, how your genes are expressed. Matthieu Ricard is the founder of Karuna-Shechen, a charitable non-profit organization rooted in the ideal of compassion in action and also an active member of the Mind and Life Institute, an organization dedicated to broadening the understanding of how the mind works by exploring the intersection between contemplative traditions and contemporary scientific inquiry. He contributes to the research on the effect of meditation on the brain at various universities in the USA and Europe. Richard J. Davidson is the William James and Vilas

Professor of Psychology and Psychiatry, Director of the Waisman Laboratory for Brain Imaging and Behaviour and the Laboratory for Affective Neuroscience. In 2006, he was awarded the first Mani Bhaumik Award by UCLA for advancing the understanding of the brain and conscious mind in healing.

The best concise description about Yoga is in 4 seminal booklets by Swami Vivekananda. The vibrant tradition further got encapsulated by Shri Aurobindo in integral Yoga. B.K.S. Iyengar demonstrated the healing effects of *huth yoga* that he took to Jayprakash Narayan and Vinoba Bhave too. Our focus is on the *Rajyoga* tradition which expounds mind-body-continuum.

The Scientific Parameters were first decided for and published by Maharishi Yogi. Through his research university, MERU (Maharishi European Research University, Switzerland). He published numerous physiological studies on the de-stressing effect of meditation that he postulated to trance and to even a quantum level. Herbert Benson from Massachusetts University, Boston came to Dharamshala to study Meditation under the mentorship of the Dalai Lama. His seminal book, '*The Relaxation Response*' (1987) was only next to that of Hans Selye's classic '*Stress of Life*' (1955). A cascade of publication in Neuroscience followed the discovery by Candane Pert of Endorphins (Molecules of Emotions, 1976). Ernest Rossi, (a friend of Dr. Vyas and co-author) took the mind body connection even to the genetic expression, (The Physiobiology of Gene Expression) and till today has studied fifteen Genes that seem to be either up or down regulated. This may be the Pinnacle of Discovering a continuity of Environment→Ideas & Thoughts→Brain→Molecules in Neurotransmission & Hormone Regulation→Cell Regulation→Genetics. The zenith of this pyramid would arrive when the final computations of Large Hadron Colider Experiment (2012) were further analyzed and taken to the next stage of experimentation.

The concept while it was practiced by Mesmer in Vienna, was simultaneously exported from India by a poor Brahmin to Paris' Abbe Faria. Only in the latter half of twentieth century did the altered state of consciousness (all meditative states are altered state of consciousness) emerge as a scientific discipline with implications for therapeutic applications. Dr. Hrishikesh Jana, a professor of physiology established a society in India, Indian Society for Clinical and Experimental Hypnosis (1976) and now they are worldwide. There are wide ranging therapeutic applications (Harvard Medical School, 2003).

Thus, though Hypnotherapy is a product of meditative process, India has very few Hypnotherapists. The fact was brought to the attention of past President of India, Dr. A.P.J. Abdul Kalam, while discussing his book '*The Family and The Nation*' which is a discourse with Acharya Mahapragya. He said that India must accelerate towards advancement of Hypnotherapy in scientific model. British Medical Association (1992) and American Medical Association (1958) have approved the therapeutic use of Hypnosis.

Baba Ramdev is spreading Meditation through mammoth public gatherings. His esoteric, mystical and almost magical cures are not a subject for scientific discussion here (Philip Lipton, *Biology of Belief*). However, Dr. Shirley Telles is engaged in in-depth scientific research that she initiated at S-VYASA and is now continuing with Baba Ramdev's scientific laboratory.

At this point Rajni interrupted me saying,

"Don't you think this is too pedantic? We are telling a story. You seem to have forgotten the point."

I replied,

"Yes, but we have to narrate our autobiography. That should include not only what we did but also what we conceived."

Rajni laughed.

"Ok. Also include that I conceived two daughters and …"

We both laughed,

"And maybe we will include their biographical contributions as well!"

Proposal

The proposal is Swami Vivekananda Institute of Stem Cell Research & Therapy and Holistic Health. At the onset it needs to be made clear that there is no contradiction in the proposal. The proposal is the pursuit of science through research and applications so as to provide a unique model for affordable health care. The institution will engage in fundamental research in stem cells and genomics. The facility will apply the proven and established science, but which is not available as yet will get the first platform, following regulatory norms laid down by ICMR. On a larger stage, keeping in Indian traditions, beginning from *Rigveda* to *Bhagavad Geeta* such as *Bahujana hitaya, bahujana sukhaya,* will be the focus (key note address Bhaskar Vyas and Roopa Dave, 2013).

After a few weeks, Geeta Jotwani from ICMR called up. She said, "Under instructions from the PMO, ICMR has constituted an expert committee to review and comment on your project. I am sending it by email as well as a hard copy." Having it sent with Geeta Jotwani, I blurted out, "Is it good? What do they say?" Geeta was short in her reply, "You will read it on your computer in a few minutes."

The letter from ICMR reads as follows,

To,
Dr. Bhaskar Vyas,
President,
Samanvaya Trust,
Parimal, Majmudarwada Raopura,
Baroda – 390001

Subject: Setting up a Stem Cell Research (Kyoto Model) and Holistic Health (SVYASA, B'Lore Model) project in a village surrounding the rural areas of VADODARA, GUJARAT.

Dear Dr. Vyas,

This has reference to your presentation to PMO ID. No. 520/31/C/108/2014-ES.2 dated 26.11.2014. The proposal was placed before the Expert Group of Stem Cell Research and Therapy. On the basis of the recommendation of the Expert Group, ICMR has the following comments to offer:

The Proposal has two components
Stem Cell Research and Therapy

Holistic Development through Meditation and Yoga

- Both the proposals are very sketchy and more of broad goals and intensions rather than specific scientific proposals for an expert review.
- There are no details of an individual project with aims, objectives, MM, anticipated outcome, division to phase 1, preclinical and phase 2, clinical, IRB clearance, etc. All this is required for a scientific review by the Expert Group.
- Expertise and experience of the investigators is not evident by their profile and their own publication in peer reviewed journals.
- It would be more appropriate if they could concentrate on one aspect of stem cell research or facility. Of all the long term goals they mentioned, Public Cord Blood banking is one promising area if they have the expertise and experience to do so. A detailed scientific proposal with the required experts could then be considered.
- Project B involves holistic care, the importance of which is now very well understood.

However, specific focus on any particular area supported by a detailed project is lacking.

This is issued with the approval of the Director General, ICMR.

Thanking you,
Dr. Geeta Jotwani.

After careful scrutiny, we understood that though there was not any criticism on the scientific merit, ICMR experts were pointing a finger to go for public cord blood banking. Soon, we received a call from Mr. S to go to the PMO with details.

Rajni and I, accompanied by Amit Goswami, went to the PMO 15 minutes before the appointed time. It was like entering the sanctum sanctorum of the temple that governs whole of India. However, it was like entering any other government office with much tighter security and we were told Mr. Silva Kumar was in a meeting with the PM that could go on for an indefinite time. We could come again the next day or wait indefinitely.

When we met Mr. S after about an hour, it was past 6 P.M. We thought he would be in a hurry to leave for home. Instead, he was well relaxed and joked that there was no scheduled closure time for the PMO.

After brief elaboration, he asked:

"Are you anywhere near discovering a new drug with stem cells?"

"A new drug discovery has not happened to India since Independence. It takes a process that may last 10 years and cost $ 130 million. Our two funded projects by the Government of India point a finger that may lead to a new drug discovery."

"You have not mentioned about holistic health in your project."

"The concept about holistic health is well formulated; therefore, it does not need elaboration. Baseline is that body and mind are intimately connected. Several conditions may be treated with hypnotherapy. Homoeopathy relies heavily on individual mindset of the patient.

Moreover, we intend to explore Ayurvedic drugs with modern scientific paradigm. This may eventually ensure Ayurvedic drugs a place with pharmacopeia of western countries."

"What can we do for you?"

"Our first requirement is land, about 10 acres. We are ready with a technology to set up a public cord blood bank facility. We have the technical know-how to set up. Both of these will need help from the state government. However, NCCS, Pune has the latest facility for cryo-preservation of cord blood derived stem cells. We will want to be updated at NCCS, Pune for a week."

We established linkage with NCCS scientist Gopal Kundu. We spent almost a whole day with Dr. Lalita Limaye, a gracious gentle lady professor willing to share knowledge. And we also came to know the erudition of Prof. Ulhas Wagh and enjoyed hospitality from ex-director G.C. Mishra. We thought that with this facilitation from the PMO, we would not only gain further insights in technology, but would also save cost. Moreover, present director at NCCS, allowed Dr. Gopal Kundu to collaborate to write a stem cell project at DBT. He asked only one question, "Why don't you do it at M.S. University?" and he was satisfied when we replied that our University had no stem cell research.

We do not know where we went wrong with NCCS this time. Their replies, formally courteous with assurance to concede to our request had a single query. We should be agreeable to pay consultation fees. We readily agreed since our perception of a consultation or observation for a few days would be around 3-4 figures. Thereafter, we were told that after careful calculation, a 5-day observation at NCCS would cost Rs. 5 lakh!

We understood that this was not a joke. Surely we must have irked or jerked someone the wrong way. The fees of this order were not unusual provided a business house was providing commercial help to another. But here the technology involved a public service: setting up a public cord blood banking facility. Prof. Lalita Limaye had mentored at length on nuances as to why one should not set up a private cord blood banking facility. Out of 45,000 samples of cord blood bank stored, there is a possibility that not more than a single child may need the stored cells. It almost amounted to exploiting a mother's love for a child that may really never need cord blood stem cells. Thus we diverted from private cord blood banking to public cord blood banking. Lalita Limaye had cautioned regarding the latter as well. There is only one public cord blood bank functioning all over the world, at New York. The reason is obvious, blood collection and blood disbursement to a patient has to be in full compliance with Helsinki declaration. It was obvious that there had to be a huge network to derive donations and funding for this project.

We did not understand why the director at NCCS, with this elementary understanding about the functioning of a public cord blood bank would have such a large commercial price. This was in sharp contradiction to their benevolent view at our earlier visit.

When we next visited the PMO, Mr. S told us that he was promoted to Finance Ministry. But, there was another IAS director, Mr. SP who was in charge. We should see him.

Mr. SP was fully aware of the previous meeting, as if we had met him personally. He inquired about NCCS and their response. When we briefed him as to what had happened, he conveyed through body-language, disbelief, annoyance and dejection. He said, "Do you have the copy of the letter?"

"Yes, here it is."

"I would like to pursue the matter, let me have a copy."

"Mr. SP, it is obvious that they do not want us to have this facilitation."

"But we would like to know why? And how they had arrived at such valuations?"

"That will further antagonize them. We have the technology and we know where else to look for verification from other academics. Kindly drop the matter."

SP closed the matter, though it was obvious he had not liked it. It may not have been open defiance but it was certainly insubordination to the highest office in the country. Such 'autonomous' behaviour will *not* set up any healthy democratic behaviour but will generate fissiparous tendencies.

Both the sides sat in silence for some time. Then we said, "Mr. SP, we leave the decision about how to act to you. We have set our course on moving straight on the stem cell matter and not on engaging in to divertive discord. Kindly oblige by understanding."

We followed up the public cord blood banking route through different agencies. Dr. Geeta Jotwani, ICMR, gave a link to go to Valsad, Gujarat. We were surprised! Valsad is a small district town that only a few years ago became a district and it has a medical college only recently established. The chief of this medical college and hospital would very likely be a senior professor who might have fallen from the grace of his higher ups and have been posted to set up the newly founded college as a punishment posting! Even if this guess was wrong, what would this professor turned administrator know about stem cells? All the same, we dropped a line that did not evoke an answer.

We gathered the information that Government of India has an ambitious plan to set up at least one public cord blood banking facility in each state of India. Quoting the reference from the

Prime Minister, we followed up with different secretaries in the Department of Health; we drew polite non-committal answers. We could not get any information about setting up public cord blood banks in every state of India. By this time we came to know that Dr. Srinivisan and Dr. Saranya had set up a public cord blood bank at Chennai as Jeevan Public Cord Blood Bank. When Government of Tamil Nadu decided to fund them with Rs. 9 crore, we decided to visit them at Chennai.

Dr. Saranya and Dr. Srinivasan had a profile that we found really attractive. Both of them were clinicians. They jettisoned their clinical career when Dr. Srinivasan sold off their pathological laboratory They succeeded to get the grant from Tamil Nadu Government as they had formulated the fees that would be very beneficial to Tamil Nadu residents.

When we landed at Chennai airport, we discovered that Chennai city had torrential rain the previous night and half the city was inundated with knee-deep water. In certain areas, fishermen provided transport with their boats! Few taxi men that were there at the airport were demanding exorbitant fares without guaranteeing to drop at the destination.

Dr. Srinivasan responded to our call congenially and said he would send a taxi to the airport. We reached Jeevan Blood Bank in about half-an-hour. There were no floods, no water on this route!

They shared the operational and technical details open-heartedly. I noted that there was a thangka hanging on the wall just above his chair. I was made to interrupt technicalities and said:

"This thangka seems to be from Tibet. We like the image of Buddha."

"No, it is from Bhutan."

"So you have been to Bhutan, for tourism?"

"No, thangka came from Bhutan to Chennai. Can you guess what would be the price?"

"Thangkas are a priceless heritage. One can buy for few thousand rupees at Tibetan markets in McLeoadganj but when preserved over centuries, as this one looks to be, the price may amount to any figure."

"Yes, this one is worth Rs. 20 lakhs!" and he laughed. Rajni and I, we were astonished.

"20 Lakhs!! How can you afford it and you have just put it in your office without being guarded!"

"In fact it is too precious to us to be priceless. It came as a blessing to us", and then he narrated the story.

A lama from Bhutan came to Chennai since he was guided to Jeevan Blood Bank. The lama was in need of hemopoietic stem cells. Jeevan found the correct match. They waived all the fees since they thought the sacred man would be penniless. When he completed the treatment with the blessings of the Almighty and left, Saranya and Srinivasan were happy to save a life and forgot about it.

One day, Dr. Srinivasan had to make a payment of Rs. 20 lakhs. The bank instalment was overdue. The resources were exhausted and no more debt was anywhere in sight. Dr. Srinivasan was feeling dejected and despondent when a lama whom he did not know arrived. He put a bundle that was wrapped in this thangka on the table. With difficulty he conveyed that this was sent as a blessing from Bhutan and briskly left. When Srinivasan unwrapped the thangka, he found that it contained Rs. 20 lakhs!

Srinivasan ran to the door. But the man had disappeared!

When amazement, wonder, surprise and astonishment about the story around the thangka and Rs. 20 lakhs slowly subsided, Rajni and I got up and bowed down to the whosoever God that the thangka symbolized. This was one more evidence that faith, genuine faith does materialize through material facts. Such instances have happened to us, though in smaller amounts, at the charitable institutions that we have founded. We were convinced that if there was one more public cord blood bank that was to survive in addition to the New York Public Cord Blood Bank, it would be Jeevan.

Saranya took Rajni to show the outlay while I continued discussions with Srinivasan. Saranya showed from first step, where cord blood in sterile container would be collected at Jeevan. There would be an aliquot that would contain about 20cc of blood to run the preliminary test. Thereafter it was almost like an assembly line processing, step-by-step. Initially red blood corpuscles would be separated and thrown out and finally, a few cc of hemopoietic stem cells would be obtained. Before storage in liquid nitrogen, human leukocyte antigen status of the cells would be verified. Dr. Saranya explained that there are 6 types of human leukocyte antigens and at least 4 of them should match with the recipient.

Srinivasan was proud to disclose that a lady professional from New York Blood Bank travelled to Chennai to set up Jeevan. He suggested that best way to collaborate would be to have another public cord blood bank at Vadodara so that the chances of finding a proper match would increase. He offered to travel to Vadodara to set up the new bank.

Here, at Jeevan, we discovered almost a clone to our self. They further welcomed a scientist from our end to be an observer, as well as Sandeep David to understand operational metrics for 2 days. It was around 4 P.M. when Srinivasan said he had to catch a flight since he had a presentation before a multinational company. They were likely to donate to Jeevan.

We reached the dining hall, Lead Bitter Chambers, Theosophical Society to find packed lunchboxes waiting for us. We looked at each other asking, "Do we need to eat more for lunch?" Both of us shook our heads and preferred to have only tea and biscuits. While eating biscuits, Rajni said,

"I have noted that they are wasting quite a few samples of cord blood."

"Well Rajni, waste is an unavoidable necessity. Rather than having inadequate number of stem cells, it is better to discard the samples altogether."

"Okay, that goes without saying. At one time, and even now, most of the blood as cord blood is thrown away. However, once it is collected in a sterile container and sent to the blood bank, the meter of the cost starts running. Do you remember that we have thought of deriving a product from the used media for culture?"

"Yes. But that was for developing a cosmetic product. How does it relate to cord blood?"

"Cord blood may be less than 100cc. I understand as an obstetrician that its collection may be the last priority when conducting a delivery. Delivery may have been through a caesarean section, in that case after the baby is handed over to the child specialist or a nurse, the cord blood should be maintaining sterility. The abdominal wound would be waiting to be closed and there may be bleeding from the uterus to be controlled before that. No wonder some of the samples would be of less than 100cc."

"But so what?"

"All the same, it will be sterile cord blood from an obviously healthy foetus. It will contain plasma proteins; both albumin and globulin. It will also contain coagulation factors. Each one of them can be a marketable product."

"Are you not having pipe dreams? Is it so easy to fractionate your products? At the moment it might appear an impossibility, but let us consult some experts in electrophoresis of proteins. Maybe from what is being considered a wastage by Jeevan, we may arrive at salvaging valuable products that support the survival of public cord blood banking."

What Rajni suggested appeared to be a genuine feminine insight. It was true for cord blood. But it was indeed feasible to fractionate plasma into various marketable products; it was being done in Surat by a classmate of mine. He had started doing it a few decades ago.

Yet another altogether novel feature to public cord blood banking emerged. One evening, Manoj Mehta, our friend in Aurobindo circle, a miracle of a survival for more than 6 years with undiagnosed cancer somewhere in his neck, attributing his survival to divine light from the Mother and Ayurvedacharya, gave us a ride back home from Aurobindo Ashram, Vadodara. He casually asked, "There is a senior Indian Institute of Management, Ahmedabad alumni who is interested to meet you. Would you like?...."

"IIM-A alumni, when interested in Shri Aurobindo, why would I not run? Is he here?"

"Though spiritual people, their agenda is not Shri Aurobindo. Along with his son, they are international businessmen. They know about your work on stem cells."

"In that case, let us meet tomorrow evening. Please confirm."

An introduction through Manoj Mehta went straight to our heart. We trusted the father and son duo, and everything they said, to the last dot. When they said that they were close to Nelson

Mandela, I jerked up and said, "Oh! I have wanted to meet him for a long, long time."

"We will make it possible. What is the most interesting story about Mandela? You might ask me to narrate his whole biography. But, to be short, I would tell a short story that *Time Magazine* published. He was invited for dinner by the Queen after assuming the office as the President. At the end of the dinner, *Time Magazine* reported that the bowls containing water with slices of lemon were served. Mandela thought this was the last drink that British would have been taking following dinner. He squeezed the lemon slices and drank it."

"Oh, that must be embarrassing!...."

"No, there was no embarrassment when Queen seated next to Mandela also followed suite and the entire gathering of guests at the table followed the Queen! I like this story for two reasons. Primarily it depicts how naively a president may behave after having spent more than 20 years in prison. Secondly, it is an epitome of diplomatic decorum by the British Queen and the guests as to how to make a prestigious guest comfortable in whatever he may do."

Finding me drawn into deep confidence, they opened up with a business proposal. A South African firm needed human red blood corpuscles from foetal blood. It was intended for pharmaceutical testing.

He continued, "We understand that you are in process of setting up a public cord blood bank."

"Your homework is only partially correct. Our blood bank is primarily for human use for larger benefit of patients. We cannot sell red blood corpuscles."

"But surely we are not asking you to sell what you are likely to process as stem cells. Whatever samples are inadequate for stem cell processing, we understand you will have to throw away. Instead, we put it to use for better pharmaceutical products. And, you would generate value out of this waste."

That our guests had done a lot of homework was easily understood. What we did not like was that they were utilizing our sensibilities to propagate business. Moreover, we faced a genuine conflict of values. Here was a proposition, if not dubious, was surely made in a rather devious way. Could we trust such a proposition? Even when it sounded fair to conduct business so that public bank could be made functional, would the means justify the end? We believed in Immanuel Kant, Aldous Huxley, Mahatma Gandhi, the Dalai Lama and Samdhong Rinpoche when they said, "The right means will lead to the right ends." We thanked the guests after a few hours and told them that we would revert back.

This is a perennial conflict, not only in dealing with stem cells, but in all other walks of our life. We have learnt to live with it since there is no resolution of this dichotomy in sight.

This feature in the proposition from the international businessmen we decided to incorporate in our write-up for public cord blood banking to be submitted to the Health Commissioner, Government of Gujarat.

Chief Secretary, Government of Gujarat and Mission Director, Gujarat State Biotechnology Mission, welcomed our idea and facilitated by setting up a meeting with the Commissioner of Medical Services, Mr. J.P. Gupta. From the onset, we sensed some reticence from Mr. Gupta. He began,

"I have addressed medical audiences of more than 500 doctors, and asked them how many of them know about stem cells. Generally, nobody raises a hand. How are you qualified to set up a public cord blood banking facility?"

We explained that stem cell science was an emerging science even in the 21st century. This was not taught at medical colleges. "We have set up a hospital for children and women. At the same hospital we have set up a blood bank that has become a premier blood bank in the state of Gujaraty" we said.

"But, cord blood banking is different from blood bank."

"Of course it is. But, the process is simple. There are already a few private cord blood banking facilities operative across the country. Storage facility is charged to the parents. About one child will benefit when 45,000 would have been stored. We consider this to be exploitation of motherhood instinct."

He showed open resentment to this activist kind of statement. He retorted.

"In that case public cord blood banking would not be cost

effective. Send me the source of the funds, for establishment and maintenance."

"Yes, this is the write up from Jeevan. We shall simply be duplicating it…."

"Alright, include that and I shall call you for a next meet after studying."

He abruptly concluded the meeting; the second call never came from Mr. J.P. Gupta. Now that there is a new incumbent in the office, probably we will pick up the thread. Maybe we did not pursue enough and persist rightfully with Mr. Gupta. Medical doctors, professors at medical college spoke well about Mr. Gupta. Most opined that he was upright and accommodating. In retrospect, we should have understood that his attitude may be because of the fact that he was being directed by the Chief Secretary. Gupta was a senior IAS officer. Though he was supposed to be subordinate to higher up, he disliked to be dictated, particularly when he was at the top of an administrative set-up.

We have been proved wrong, once again, about land allocation. We presumed that being recommended by the Prime Minister's Office would make allocation a smooth sailing. The belief got fortified when the Chief Secretary, Government of Gujarat, called us for a 1-to-1 meet and instructed the Collector, Vadodara, to facilitate. Only later we understood that the special meeting with the Chief Secretary was a mischance. His secretary had thought us to be in multi-crore category of investors.

We generally give a pass to sordid encounters. But this one is so difficult to forget. Frankly putting it across as facilitation money, not only for himself, but that would surely percolate all the way higher up to Gandhinagar, a minion of an officer wanted 98 lakhs! We asked him, "You are putting the message straight, in blunt and blatant words. Should you not be a bit bashful?"

"I was so once upon a time when I worked as a small government servant. I was used as a conduit. I had to stand before the bosses to whom I delivered. I was constantly afraid that, not only did I risk my job but could be sent to jail also."

"That's right. What was wrong in thinking that way?"

"I discovered a right way. I resigned from my job. By this time,

I had a data pool of almost all the pieces of land in this taluka. I knew *jantri*—ongoing government rate—on my lips. I would also tell ongoing market rates just by counting on my fingertips. This was the business acumen that I had. I set up a single room office. My business, I categorize as consulting advice.

I further found out a way to derive respect. I have been elected as a village panchayat member. So, I am now being offered a chair at every meeting that I'm supposed to attend."

There was no point in arguing with this successful businessman that his logic was perverted. We decided to change the track, and opted for a piece of land at a different location.

For over 5 years, we followed up with 3 collectors, District Development Officer, District Health Officer, Mamlatdars and Talatis at Vadodara. The process is still on and we never gave up hope. Though the process is arduous and not without sordid experiences, hope lies eternal in our breast.

13

Nobody can Deny an Idea Whose Time has Come: Regulations will Come and Go

Clear out the entire forest: but cut not a single tree. So said J. Krishnamurti. We would like to say, let quackery and quacks be entirely eliminated, but let not a single patient be denied who may benefit from stem cell therapy.

Political pundits concur across the globe that the government that governs the least is the best form of government. Karl Marx dreamt of a utopian state of dictatorial governance where *state shall wither away*!

Howsoever transparent a process and regardless of numerous checks and counter-checks, a sanction to perform is issued at a window with a single sentry-signatory. A higher up at the helm of the affairs, when out of office revealed the secret to us with a wily smile, let everyone vote for the favour of a resolution; let the entire executive body rectify. I know that it can be executed only with my signature. When to sign is not enshrined in any constitution!

Former Vice President of USA, Spiro Theodore Agnew, was bribed by a businessman for a mere $10000! The businessman, while walking out of Vice President's office was 'shaking in his boots' and ran to the media to clear his conscience. *Time* magazine quoted the businessman "I asked myself what I am doing? I am bribing the second most powerful man in the world." Agnew had to resign. A Japanese Prime Minister, Kakuei Tanaka, when caught in a similar act defended himself that it is customary in Japanese tradition to accept a return for a favour.

Charismatic Indian Prime Minister, Indira Gandhi, defended corruption as a global phenomenon. When her son Rajiv Gandhi became Prime Minister, he said that only 15 paisa per rupee percolates down to the beneficiary granted by the government.

We have had a rare privilege to sit across R. Venkataraman at Chennai, after his retirement from Presidential Office. We were on our annual retreat at Theosophical Society in Adyar, Chennai. The appointment was readily granted. We reached his residence prepared to wait for the appointment. We were pleasantly surprised to see the waiting area empty.

The office of the previous President of India was about 12 by 12 square feet. There was an office table of about 6 feet by 3 feet. There was 1 executive chair and 3 poorly carved out wooden chairs across the table. Yes, there were some decorations; a flower vase on the table with a few freshly plucked flowers.

He was radiating benevolence from his face. He inquired amicably about the hospital for the inauguration of which he had come to Vadodara. His face gleamed a bit more when we mentioned about Gopal Gandhi, his personal secretary at that time. He asked, whether we had known the latest news about Gopal Gandhi, as he had recently taken over as Governor of West Bengal. After some time, the secretary entered the room and we realized that our time is over. So we stood up and requested for an autograph on the book, 'My Presidential Years'.

He was obviously more pleased and said, "Of course I will sign it. Have you read the book?"

We had read the review in 'The Hindu'. He carried on talking disregarding the fact that our allocated time was up.

"The chapter concerning the mercy petition following the death sentence awarded to the assassin Kehar Singh."

"Why?"

"The chapter portrays poignantly, a conflict in the conscience of the then President of India. The President is known to be a generously kind hearted person. He would have been inclined to grant the mercy petition. While the chapter describes that the president has to be guided by the legalities that are involved, we understand that you may also have had a few sleepless nights."

"No, I always sleep well, since I conscientiously do my duty and do not worry about the consequences."

During the conversation, he asked us to sit down. Finding him even more relaxed with the personal notes, I ventured to ask him, "Sir, during your long tenure in the office, you may have come across different kinds of people. Did you have any experience; may I use the word 'encounter', with somebody offering grease money?"

"I entered politics at a time when Gandhian ideals were still paramount. My image as a puritan was well known across India. My wife, Janki, (when she travelled to Dwarka in an unreserved compartment) was publicised as religious wife of a sanctimonious husband. But, the Japanese did not know this.

They even put pressure that not to accept a return gift is considered a violation of Japanese tradition. I replied to them to add one more piece of the item that they are selling to Indian government as a gift."

"But sir, now generations have passed. Times have changed."

R. Venkataraman closed the discussion by saying, "I see corruption for kickback or whatever name you may call it, as a matter for the personal attitude of an individual. Our heritage is fundamentally based on *sanatan dharma. Dharma* is a way of life. Of course, people will live their life as per their own choice."

Before leaving the premises, I went over to the personal secretary and thanked him. I said "You have facilitated a memorable instance in our lives. Now may I ask some more facilitation?"

I continued "We have made confirmed railway reservations before leaving Vadodara. Now we are told that Chennai office had not received any such message. The coaches are fully booked; therefore, they are not able to help us. Will you please help with VIP quota?"

"Of course. You have been our guests. But even otherwise I utilize this facility for several others."

At the railway station, we approached the coach conductor. He looked at the tickets and said, "Oh, VIP quota. How is Venkataraman sir?"

"He is fine and the gentleman president is still serving the nation."

"Yes, only the other day, I saw him on TV addressing a gathering at Krishnamurti Foundation."

As the train started, to our surprise, the supposedly fully booked coach had several berths vacant. Rajni asked, "What is this?" showing the vacant berths.

"The nuances and the metrics of this situation are difficult to decipher. Maybe other seats reserved for VIP quota were not occupied. Waitlisted passengers would have cancelled as we were about to cancel. But rather than mulling over such problematic solutions, let us travel comfortably back to Vadodara."

Rajni asked rather sarcastically and half-jokingly, "Would you not call this corruption?"

"You ask the railway minister for an answer. What we have done is entirely legal and no grease money is paid."

We laughed.

When we decided to leave USA in 1969 it was said to be the year of the gold rush in USA. We had consciously decided to be conscientious that only need and never any greed will be a driving force in our lives.

So as a small private enterprise, engaged in fundamental research, we had thought that we will not have anything to do with governmental agencies. Our initial contact with government officials went really smooth as discussed earlier. Mr. Shashikumar from Department of Biotechnology had assured us that New Delhi is really new in the 21st century.

An imperative arose when we decided to apply funding from Government of India agencies. A beneficiary to receive the grant has to have recognition from Department of Science and Industrial Research. Both the scientists working with us at that time were repugnant to write an application. I would have conceded to their dislike. But I gathered up myself to prepare a hasty draft and sent it online. But there happened to be a candid talk on the telephone. The voice said, "I am Mr. Deshpande from DSIR. We would like to invite you for a personal presentation."

"Mr. Deshpande, thank you, but I am under heavy workload."

"We will facilitate you to schedule a date for presentation."

I paused. What does he mean? I went informal and said, "You will be a lifesaver. I am to visit New Delhi for an ICMR sponsored symposium. Can you give me a slot during any of the two days?"

"For sure, Dr. Vyas, please come at 12 noon on the very first day."

ICMR had sponsored a two day workshop with the title, "Stem Cell Therapy: Hope or Hype". In her keynote, Prof. Vatsala indicated the trend that the workshop is likely to gravitate towards hyperbolic claims for therapy with stem cells. I wondered, where is she leading to? But we left to rush for DSIR presentation.

Contrary to the expectations at reception at a government office, I was told that Mr. Deshpande would ask for me after a few minutes since a presentation earlier than mine was in progress.

It was a large hall that would have accommodated around 500 people. I waited at a distance. The earlier presenters left from a side door. I had to wait for a few more minutes till a man rushed past, hurriedly shook hands with Mr. Deshpande and shortly thereafter I was called. Mr. Deshpande began with a conciliatory note. "Your research is on stem cells. So I have called the gentleman from ICMR to be present as well."

I requested help to set up my laptop screen to connect to the projector. Gentleman from ICMR willingly complied. It was like an examiner facilitating a candidate.

I presented a brief that we had prepared for Varshney at Gujarat Venture Finance Ltd.

Mr. Deshpande then asked, "What are your publications for stem cell research?"

"Between 2 promoters, we have more than 50 publications in the respective areas of our disciplines."

"How many of them are for stem cell research?"

"We have yet to begin with our research."

"The department expects that researchers should have at least one publication in the area of dedicated research before granting research status."

"We shall soon publish."

ICMR representative asked, "What innovations have you made in the form of devices?"

"We have devised a contraption by which we transport stem cells from Vadodara to Pune."

"That is not an innovation. Such transportations are a routine."

Within a short time, we were informed that our present status does not justify for research recognition by DSIR. However, we were advised to apply with at least one publication.

Though I had not wanted any recognition, having been denied it spurred me on. This took me to a conference in Bhubaneswar.

We prepared a research paper on how the metaphoric semantics in altered states of consciousness may change genetic expression. We have thought for long on the subject and published papers in collaboration with Ernest Rossi. So as to save time for publication in a research journal, we sent the research papers to the Society for Translational Research that was to hold their biannual meet at Bhubaneswar.

Dr. Bharat Aggarwal, chairman, conveyed the acceptance promptly. Journey to Bhubaneswar was a much delayed wish fulfilment. Konark Sun Temple utilizes a wheel as a symbol to represent the journey that the Sun God takes day after day. Thus wheel has symbolized time in Hindu Tradition. We have been enamoured with this similar metaphor in Buddhist tradition too. At most Buddhist temples, rotating wheels are displayed. What the devotees may understand about rotating a wheel as a symbol of time does not need to be even questioned. The symbolic meaning to a select few will give a semantic translation to the Wheel of Time. The rest are happy to have paid reverence to a time honoured symbol. So it turned out to be a *Yatra* as well.

Prof. Pathak Sen, Professor of Genomics at M.D. Anderson, Texas, who presided at the time of presentation came across after the session and we sat together for some time. I had made a statement that, "In altered state of consciousness such as meditation, relaxation response, hypnosis and other varieties of religious experiences etc. (which might collectively grouped as State of *Turya;* consciousness), the words expand to a semantic transformation so that virtual may be seen as Real."

He said that, "I am a firm believer that meditation and such states do make an impact on genomics. Such research is underway at our centre. This is increasingly recognized by the West." He was highly interested with research in Ayurveda and he had invited Baba Ramdev to demonstrate *Hath-Yoga* practices to their centre in USA. He showed interest to collaborate to apply for funding. Although the desired collaboration did not materialize, this instance poignantly shows how the quest for stem cell research can translate into genomics.

Thus I thank DSIR for the *Yatra* to Bhubaneswar. We reapplied to DSIR having published this article. Deshpande promptly replied that we need not travel to Delhi as he will soon be visiting Vadodara. He will let us know the dates.

Howsoever hospitable we may try to be, our perceptions with guests have generally turned out to be at variance. We had written to Deshpande that he will be our guest at a hotel nearby. He had accepted. He was received at the hotel and we all had a pleasant dinner.

But a catastrophe was waiting the next morning. Mr. Deshpande was to leave by evening flight back to Delhi. After the inspection, we had organized a sightseeing tour for him. When Nirupa went to pick him up, she deposited his bag at the reception. She then left with Mr. Deshpande to bring him to the stem cell facility. When Mr. Deshpande realised that this meant that he would be billed only for a night's stay he became very agitated.

Deshpande paused, looked sternly at Nirupa. "No, No, No. How can you touch my bag without my permission? My department pays me two days charges and I pay the bill. I do not accept this. Please turn the car and put the bag in my room where it was!"

Nirupa did what she was ordered to do. Lucky the same room was still vacant. Hotel staff understood the metrics. They assured they will prepare a separate bill etc.

When they arrived, Mr. Deshpande was taken for the inspection by Rajni. Taking me aside, Nirupa briefed me what had happened. I wondered if this would be taken badly by Mr. Deshpande. We swiftly moved on with the presentation. He had only a few questions:

"Where is your stem cell manufacturing facility?"

"The manufacturing facility will be set up at about 20 miles from here at Biotech Park, Savli. Would you like to visit it?"

"No."

"Have you imported any appliances and machinery?"

"No and even if DSIR recognition will facilitate customs duty exemptions etc., we are committed to the ideal, 'Be Indian, Buy Indian'. We will not want to buy an imported facility, even if it turns out to be cheaper."

We then invited him to join us for lunch at our home.

He accepted and we dared to relax. We felt we were within touching distance of winning.

Mr. Deshpande spent an hour after lunch with a post graduate from the University who wanted guidance from him. The project had a plan to extract fibre like material from sugarcane waste which could then be made into sanitary pads. Deshpande approved and asked him to go ahead with his research product. He was willing to help. We parted on amicable terms.

After a few days, Deshpande called to say that DSIR was granting approval for three instead of two years. We thanked him.

At our next visit, we went personally to DSIR to thank Mr. Deshpande. The man in his chair, Mr. Rao said, "Deshpande Sir has retired some time back. Gentleman that he was, we miss him for his kindness and clean dealings. But I am aware about you. If you need any help, please call, you need not take the trouble to travel to New Delhi.

We had not anticipated even in our dreams that we would need to take the help of the DSIR before the three years were up. But within a short time, another storm blew over that began with SBIRI application already granted!

About three years before this event, Government of Gujarat had announced an ambitious plan to host a biotech park at Savli, near Vadodara. They had acquired hectares of land. The park was to be developed in three phases. As part one, a magnificent office building was erected. The most enticing part of the scheme was an incubator. That meant that most of the expensive equipments needed were to be housed there and would be available for use as an outsourcing means. A mission director with spacious offices and a couple of executives were supposed to be functional. As discussed in the earlier chapters, we were the first to apply for 1 hectare of land. We were also the first to be allotted and we immediately paid up Rs. 20 lakhs to become the first allottee to be handed over the plot. We dug up the tube-well to draw water and, a small cottage was built to store masonry equipment.

But there was no sign of an incubator being developed. One could only see some donkeys grazing around there. On periodic visits, our scientist (who took her young toddler with her) would report that her son had a free ride on the donkey and that some of the masonry tools were being pilfered away. When we complained this to the mission director, he referred us to the Collector, Vadodara. The Collector promptly replied that the plot being in our possession, its security was our responsibility. "If you like, you complain to the police." Thus the time elapsed by. Instead of erecting a compound wall, we planted trees along the proposed fence. It was a pleasure to see them growing tall rapidly in this fertile, barren land.

A few months before the completion of 3 years following allotment of land to us, we got a notice from the executive engineer of GIDC. He drew our attention to the fact if we do not develop the stem cell facility before completion of 3 years, the land will be confiscated back by the government. We had not known this stipulation before this notice arrived. We approached the mission director. He agreed that they had not been able to develop the incubator. Hence, the directive was modified to say that the government will take back the land, but will pay back the cost of the land plus an added interest of 6 per cent.

We persisted with the mission director that providing incubator facility was a promise which they could not renegade on. We were being pressurized by the land allocation authority (GIDC) for the return of the land. I wrote a letter saying that I would not return the land and in case of litigation, would cite GSBTM to have a collateral responsibility.

Only then an executive from GSBTM came to met us. We would like to believe that he was a Good Samaritan. He advised that any litigation apart from long proceedings will put us in a grey zone with the government. Some people at GSBTM may lose their jobs. Another company in a situation similar to ours, has succeeded in selling off their company altogether. GSBTM will have no objection to a similar repeat by us. We were amazed at the win-win situation.

Finding a buyer proved very difficult. The price of the land had rocketed. The only proposed development could be that related to stem cell. Moreover, the land itself could not be sold.

We were almost in a rat-trap. It was our good fortune that an entrepreneur in pharmaceutical business needed the land. They ingeniously suggested a solution. The land cannot be sold: but the company that owns the land can certainly sell itself. Our company had developed research products and applied for government grants. These were the only assets of our stem cell company—Total Potential Cell. We divided our company into two segments. One segment was tagged to the Savli land and sold. We retained the other segment and named it 'Total Potential Cells.'

We frequently asked ourselves: "Does this not amount to a break of contract, does it not mean cheating, is this a criminal offence?" We invoked Saibaba too. Did he answer? We do not know. But we considered this as a SOS situation. The legal experts were absolutely sure that a company can sell out itself. The buyer buys the assets with full understanding of the liabilities. That was a win-win situation. The deal went through and now a large factory operates at this site.

Soon after we were granted the first research project on stem cells by Small Business Innovation Research Initiative-SBIRI. A team comprising of two eminent experts and one financial and business advisor visited us for due diligence. Scientific experts were obviously pleased.

Shortly thereafter, the first instalment of the grant money was deposited in the bank account of 'Total Potential Cells Pvt. Ltd.'

We informed DSIR about changing the name of our company. They did not seem too interested. "We understand that in business there can be various reasons for a turnabout. That does not concern us. As long as the same people are doing the same research, we are not inclined to investigate further."

We carried on with our research work. However, fate had other plans and we ran into stormy weather once again....

We were allotted a further grant titled 'Biotechnology Ignition Grant.' Managing Director of Biotechnology Industry Research Assistance Council-BIRAC visited our laboratory for due diligence.

We sat along with Prof. Bharat Chattoo at Genome Research Centre, M.S. University for few hours to finalise our presentations. All the dots and dashes were verified. Just as we thought we had finished, the managing director said, "You have mentioned that you have been granted a SBIRI project. That does not reflect on our records." Promptly, we dashed out the grant disbursement papers. She put them in her file and we thought the matter had ended. A short time after, we had a letter from business executive from BIRAC, Mr. Das. The letter was tersely worded. It said, "There are serious discrepancies between the two applications for grant. SBIRI grant was accorded to 'Total Potential Cell.' BIG grant is being processed for 'Total Potential Cells'. Both the companies are different." A copy was sent to Prof. Bharat Chattoo since he was a collaborator.

Anybody who would have read the matter for the first time would have thought that we were up to some swindling. When we met Prof. Bharat Chattoo, he was obviously agitated. He could not hide his annoyance and asked, "Bhaskarbhai, what is this? How could you have done this?"

We pacified the professor and reassured him that there was no swindling whatsoever. We explained the circumstances whereby we had to sell off the company at Biotech Park, Savli. The grants were awarded to the research branch that was separately located as per the rules. The grant money was being utilized for the purpose of same research on mesenchymal stem cells by the same research team.

Prof. Bharat Chattoo then called up the managing director, BIRAC. He assured her that there was no *mala fide*. Should she desire, we would personally go to BIRAC, New Delhi, to explain. She said she was satisfied but wanted the explanation in writing. The business executive, who had written some scornful accusations softened his outlook. The BIG grant was released. Mr. Rao, at DSIR, also renewed the research recognition with the revised name of the company.

Rajni and I, once again met Mr. Rao to thank him. He was eloquently elaborate this time. He said, "Howsoever well meaning a government servant maybe, he has to be constantly aware that he is walking on a razor's edge. He narrated a story of a Delhi transport bus conductor who was found guilty. He had pilfered small change by issuing a smaller denomination ticket than the money collected. The conductor had 29 years of service. He lost not only the job, but the pension rights etc. as well."

He emphasized that, had the government agencies, SBIRI, BIRAC and DBT not conceded to our representation, he would certainly not take the risk.

We understood.

Fortunately, the storm has blown over.

Both the funded projects have yielded results that have a potential for developing new drugs/therapies for diabetes and osteoarthritis. At the baseline, we have succeeded in establishing that stem cells have the property of translation to all three germinal layers. These cells would undergo translation to the tissue type of the cell that may be needing regeneration.

Further, an autobiography should end just before the writer is about to die. But is not dead. In my instance, the autobiography continues with a self-volunteered message to the researchers and many more sufferers with no kind of therapy available to them. I had peripheral neuritis as a complication of type 2 diabetes. All the nerves from head to toe were giving me kind of electrical shocks. Vitamin B-1 supplements and most powerful analgesics failed to provide relief. Thereafter, I resorted to stem cell therapy. At that time, even the consent of compassionate approval was not in vogue.

Necessity is the mother of invention. There will be situations where a precious person in an erudite stem cell research oriented family will have no established line of treatment. In that instance, family, friends and the patient himself would like to be treated with stem cells, regardless of the fact that current rules would not allow this treatment. We are assured that stem cell application will be available in India and most researchers will provide benefit, at least to the extent of 25 per cent of improvement. That is the general consensus.

Indian Council of Medical Research came into existence before Independence. The institution is comparable to the Papacy at Vatican. The Pope is satisfied with having proclaimed 10 commandments that prohibit practice of some vices that should be the way for religious heads; one would have expected that ICMR will promote and facilitate research with positive strokes. A monolithic structure and several committees that dart to and fro across India is the only sign of research development at ICMR.

About 50 years back, we had published a research paper about the stress response in burn patients. The clinical significance was that patients with very high stress response index had a poor prognosis. We felt we have achieved a pinnacle of success when this was published in the *ICMR Journal.*

Hence, we hold ICMR in high regard. We tried to collate with at least 2 extramural research institutions that are being funded by ICMR grant. We cannot name the institutions since the researchers frankly admitted that, 'who cares for their research?' It was submitted to the parent body ICMR, and it may be lying in some forlorn corner in a multi-storeyed building.

India has a population that is burgeoning with leaps and bounds year after year. India has yet to produce a single new drug. Stem cell science has proven that there are regenerative properties in mesenchymal stem cells. The applications can be vast and varied.

When we read 2006 edition of guidelines for research and therapy for stem cells by ICMR, we were pleased. What leniency! What flexibility! How easily doable again and again! M.S. University has numerous faculties in biological sciences. There are eminent clinicians as professors at Medical College, Vadodara. We believe professors have high erudition and ethics. We carefully read the eligibility criteria for being a member of the Institutional Committee for Stem Cell Research. We appreciated the wisdom in excluding the promoters and investigators of the research from being members of the committee. Instead, we personally exhorted the committee members to be our conscience keepers.

We put the relevant literature support on the table. We circulated the guiding principles enunciated at Helsinki.

Thus, we felt that our Institutional Committee for Stem Cell Research will be accorded recognition. Thereafter, selecting an area of research where we have established the proof of concept will naturally follow with an approval from National Apex Committee for Stem Cell Research and Therapy (NAC-SCRT).

But we were in a fool's paradise. We had no understanding of the science concerning the functioning of 'commitology'.

We received a brief communication from Dr. Vijay Kumar, Secretary, NAC-SCRT, informing us that NAC has not approved the constitution of our institutional committee for stem cell research. No reasons were assigned. However, it was mentioned that we should reapply again.

Anant Marathe and I approached Vijay Kumar at ICMR. When we knocked and entered the room, a gentleman sitting on the front table typing on a typewriter said, "Hello!"

Introducing ourselves, we said, "We have come to meet Dr. Vijay Kumar, Secretary."

Congenially, he said, "I am Vijay Kumar! What can I do for you?"

Showing the letter to him, we said, "We have received this letter from you. We need guidance, what should we do next?"

"Dr. Vyas, I am a secretary to some 800 committees at ICMR, would you believe that such a secretary will have time to look after your company? I can tell you, I have no inclination to follow up. Surely, do carry on your research. My colleague, Dr. Geeta Jotwani will guide you...."

"Yes, we have known Dr. Geeta. We shall go to her."

The informal conversation could have been a dialogue between college mates. All three of us remained standing in the ante room. Pleasantly surprised and pleased with this kind of demeanour from Dr. Vijay Kumar, we approached Dr. Geeta Jotwani.

Anant Marathe met Dr. Geeta Jotwani for the first time. An elegant professional lady, courteous yet, certainly no nonsense, perfect professional etiquette. She met us in her small office. Just as we were beginning to talk, Dr. Geeta excused herself to answer a phone call on the landline. We could not identify the caller, but Dr. Geeta told off the man across the line, "Do not make such calls again. I repeat, do not call again!" and she put the phone down.

Anant Marathe and I exchanged glances but Geeta Jotwani was a formally courteous lady. I asked, "Dr. Geeta, we just met Dr. Vijay Kumar, since we got a letter from him. This was a surprise. Usually you have been writing to us."

"Dr. Vijay Kumar is the Member-Secretary of NAC-SCRT. I am a member, but I am here to help."

She held a hardcopy of stem cell guidelines and patiently explained to us. The principal investigators and co-principal investigators of any project cannot be the members of the Institutional Committee for Stem Cell Research. A few times in between, Anant Marathe received numerous messages on his mobile. Finally, Dr. Geeta conveyed brisk annoyance by turning her face in the other direction. Anant Marathe understood and he switched off his phone.

Meanwhile I argued with Dr. Jotwani, "But, we should at least be accorded a recognition for the constitution of ICSCR."

Geeta concluded, "It is up to the committee."

Once we were out of the room, having walked a few steps away, Anant Marathe ensured that nobody could hear us. He then exclaimed, "What a formidable woman, sorry not a woman, a lady!"

I mused in my mind. No wonder Anant Marathe is saying this! I said, "We were recanting 12 names of powerful masculine Sun God. Do you remember?"

"Yes, of course. But that was before a presentation that we had to make. What about that now?"

"Praying to 12 different forms of Sun God yielded splendid rewards for us. Devi Lalita has 1000 names to her various forms. One formidable form of this feminine Devi is Durga. When pleased, she can demolish even giant demons to protect a devotee. It is better that one does not brush against such a formidable form of Devi Druga !"

Yes, yes, yes. Both of us concurred.

I had known Dr. Alok Srivastava, haematologist at Christian Medical College, Vellore. He was affable at a conference. So I called him up on the phone. This time, when I identified myself as a researcher in Mesenchymal stem cells, his response was contemptuous, and indignant. He said, "Mesenchymal stem cells? Yes, we could have talked on haemopoietic stem cell research. But, so far, I have not dirtied my hands with mesenchymal stem cells!" And he cut the conversation.

I reported the matter to Prof. Bharat Chattoo. We thought he may have known Alok Srivastava. Instead he voiced reciprocal contempt, "When he says 'he has not dirtied his hands with MSC', how does he justify being the chairman?"

Thereafter, year after year after year we reapplied for recognition of ICSCR. There was a stereotype rejection signed by Dr. Vijay Kumar. After every rejection, Dr. Geeta Jotwani patiently helped us to reconstitute with suitable members. At one of such meetings, Rajni and I showed her grant letters from Department of Biotechnology. At that time, Dr. Geeta brightened up with a sparkle on her face. We thought, this time we would get our recognition. Moreover, eminent professorial scientists, such as Dr. Ramesh Bhonde, Dr. Ulhas Wagh, Dr. Ramchandran and Dr. Bharat Chattoo were also the members.

Instead, we were astonished to come across news briefing made by Dr. Geeta Jotwani on behalf of ICMR. This was flashed across most English and Hindi media newspapers. There was a photograph of Geeta Jotwani as well. It said on the headline, 'Stem cell therapy punishable with 2 years imprisonment. Medical licence to be forfeited for the stem cell therapist.'

However, an option was given for genuine researchers. They were advised to report their research to ICMR with successful results.

Needless to say, most clinicians saw such an invitation as a death threat. Who would want to jump into such a deep well? When we discussed with our friends and well-wishers, that we will respond, their response was: "Fools jump in where angels fear to tread." But such an adage was no deterrent to what we have done and that too with genuine research which had achieved favourable results.

I called up Dr. Geeta Jotwani. In a laconic mode, I asked her that she may revoke my medical licence but please she may not put me in prison, life would be hard over there. When I further asked how many replies the ICMR had received, she hesitatingly said only one!

We did not understand at that time that we were having a myopic view. ICMR attitude was generated over a panoramic span of last few years. In 2007, ICMR had held a national conference inviting stem cell participants from across the country. The title of the conference was, 'Stem Cell Therapy: A Hope or A Hype?' At this conference, speaker after speaker presented negative results; except Dr. Habibullah from Hyderabad. This was marginalized as an exception, even though he had reported pluripotent stem cell as a substitute for liver transplant. In concluding remarks, Dr. Vatsala, Chairman, certainly showed bias towards hype rather than a hope.

Thereafter, ICMR convened meetings of stem cell stakeholders in 4 major cities across India beginning from Delhi. Dr. Geeta Jotwani was the convener. She steered the discussion to highlight the newly framed guidelines for research. She emphasized therapy is proven only for haemopoietic stem cells. Once again, we had misinterpreted this gesture as facilitating the researchers. It was aimed at building a prejudiced stance towards MSCs. By this time, there were several centres across the country providing MSC for neuro-restoration and such other conditions. Most of them had tried to walk along the dotted guidelines. They had found the doors locked at NAC-SCRT. Several clinicians thereafter decided to walk along on their own. There was immense literature support across the globe concerning stem cell research including Mesenchymal Stem Cells.

It appears that not only the conscience of ICMR would have been hurt, but multinational pharmas were also against the development of stem cell therapy. Political leverage was exercised. Politicians in power were making statements against stem cell therapy. Only thereafter, ICMR has warned through national newspapers about punishing the clinical doctors. Had it not been for the then Drug Controller General of India, Dr. Ramteke, stem cell research in India would have been thrown into a blind alley. Ramteke had dared to state that he was under tremendous political pressure in a letter that was put in public domain.

We had a chance meeting with Ramteke at a BIRAC Conference in Delhi. When we warmly congratulated him, he was politely humble. He was doing his duty as required by the protocol. But the colleague, sitting next to him went on to explain that Ramteke was about to retire in a few months. Had the party in power been re-elected, Ramteke would not have been forgiven and may have even lost his pension.

Ramteke sat mutely smiling. At the conclusion, he simply said, "Men may come and men may go. Institutions last for ever. My small contribution as a Director of Drug Control would be that I have stopped the practice of pharmaceutical heads dictating their terms to the Drug Control office altogether." The directorate now is completely digitised. Drug trials are to be submitted online and are immediately notified as 'in process'.

In a democratic system, public policy, we came to understand, is in a continuous emerging process. There has got to be checks and counter-checks. Till the process has become a well connected metric with interconnections, so far so good. Instead, when the interacting agencies confront each other with ego problems, it tends to be dangerous. A baby may also be thrown with the bathwater. A government that governs the least is the best form of government. But that is not a purview for the politicians. Their lifespan lasts between two elections. With a few exceptions, when politicians emerge as statesmen, most of the crowd is busy making hay when the sun shines. Public administration is mostly subservient. Their eyes are glued to promotions and pensions. Only a microscopic minority will dare to be defiant. While it may be argued that the other pillars of good governance such as the judiciary and media will maintain balance, we came to understand that the future of small entrepreneurs like us is at a high risk, when treading an uncharted path. Therefore, it is simple: Why risk with innovations? We have a simple answer. There is an itch that is difficult to control—creative itch.

The innovative minority amongst human beings is estimated to be about 2 per cent. While we consider ourselves to be fortunate amongst this minority group, most of our fellows and friends consider this group to be crazy.

When dialogue and debate generates a conflict, not between small stakeholders like entrepreneurs, but between well defined authorities, it is a sign of good omen. ICMR is an autonomous body. Drug Control Authority is a well stipulated authority of over 100 years. In 2017, DCGI decided to consider Stromal Vascular Factor as a drug. The matter was put in public domain. Only one agency objected, ICMR! Reconciliation was provided by including stem cells as a drug. ICMR, DCGI and several stakeholders with small researchers are in a win-win situation with this inclusion. We are now assured that the revocation of medical licence and imprisonment will fall into a forgotten category.

Our pursuit of approval by NAC-SCRT went on relentlessly year after year. Soumya Swaminathan took over as the Director of ICMR after the post remained vacant for a long time. We heaved a sigh of relief. We had met Prof. Swaminathan, the father of Green Revolution in India, at a conference in Hyderabad. When we took a young farmer from Saurashtra, Gujarat, to introduce to the professor of genomics, we had found a really congenial, nationalist to the core person willing to help young, budding agriculturists. Prof. Swaminathan spent quite some time inquiring about the modified genomics of wheat that not only increases the yield but also increases the protein content up to 15 per cent. He even acknowledged that he has read about this research, as certified by Wheat Research Institute of India. He had asked the farmer, "Are you the same farmer, how did you reach the front page of the *Economic Times*?

We wrote about this story to Dr. Soumya. We requested for a meeting at ICMR, Delhi. When we got a prompt appointment, our hopes for NAC recognition went high.

This was indeed precious. We thought this might be a final breakthrough to the deadlock that we had been encountering for a long time. My tendency is to drop my guard when I see a congenial, friendly person across the table. This may be acceptable when nothing is to be bartered. Here there was a motivation to get something that we desired. So, we included Amit Goswami to be a conscientious observer at the meet.

Finding Dr. Geeta Jotwani in attendance with the Director was an additional bonus. Dr. Geeta gave a broad smile of welcome and recognition.

We exchanged pleasantries whilst tea and snacks were served. We elaborated our connections with ICMR. As a medical college teacher, Rajni was awarded a grant for PAP smear testing. Rajni had reported that it was too expensive to be used as a screening test for mass population.

Dr. Soumya smiled and said, "So you have saved national wastage. In my research on tuberculosis, we have saved several precious lives with early diagnostics by mass screening." She looked at me and asked, "What about you?"

"I have published my research findings on stress parameters in burns, way back in 1965. Recently, we sent a research for publication to *ICMR Journal*. Unfortunately it remained unpublished."

Soumya Swaminathan was surprised, "Why?"

Amit Goswami's face suddenly looked stern when I was about to open my mouth that the article was about stem cell research as a therapy for osteoarthritis, instead I swallowed a gulp. Everyone understood that this is not to be discussed at the first meeting. I reminded myself that we had decided to let the relationship develop first.

Regardless of congeniality and hospitality from Dr. Soumya Swaminathan, our homework failed. Some time later, she opted to migrate to the USA. Of course, our hopes were denied and we were left disappointed. We had thought that Dr. Soumya would be a patriotic daughter. Her father's research had ensured that India became a rice exporting nation. Following this Prof. Swaminathan had numerous offers to work outside India. He had refused to emigrate and spent his working life in India.

We have wondered what would be the reason for Soumya Swaminathan to leave for USA. The answer is difficult to guess since women have various roles to perform along with being a professional. Dr. Soumya had worked hard to climb a highly competitive ladder. To be Director at the autonomous ICMR was a pinnacle of success. Along with the perks of her professional job, there were numerous domestic perks available as well.

The salary as WHO would definitely be better. Would this have been the reason she emigrated? Rajni and I would like to believe that motherly form of Devi Lalita, Soumya, would have prevailed. We trust Soumya Swaminathan as *Ya devi sarva bhuteshu, matru rupena sang sthita.... !* So Rajni and I pray that professional Soumya has also found personal happiness.

We decided to probe with a different mode. The aim was to preempt any action by the surveillance agencies. We, therefore, wrote to Central Drugs Standard Control Organisation and Drug Controller General of India and invited them to inspect our laboratory. In the request letter, at the end, I wrote, 'Please be our conscience keeper and surely point out whatever mistake we may have made!'

We thought that we had bypassed ICMR! Much to our astonishment, the four member team that arrived for inspection included Geeta Jotwani as the ICMR representative. At the doorstep, Dr. Geeta took Nirupa aside and whispered in her ear, "I have a conflict of interest with other members of the team!"

In our inimitable style, we instructed our scientists to provide full disclosure. At one point, the chief of the team started to grill our scientists. One of them ran over to me in another room and said, "We need help."

When I saw that the questioning had an ulterior motive, I went to the chief of the team and said, "Sir, your name connotes with Bhagwan Shiva. I am in a full disclosure mode, so I say that I have direct relationship with Lord Shiva, the Kailasapati. I worship him. Please find further faults and make sure that they are on the record."

No wonder that the team was not pleased. They did find 2 or 3 small technical points for not renewing the contracts for maintenance etc. Thereafter we have not tried to walk into the lion's den voluntarily. At some discomfiture, at long last, we have come to understand that discretion is better than valour!

14

Conference at Jawaharlal Nehru University, New Delhi: Collaboration with King's College of London

One fine day on a sunny winter morning, Professor Pranav Desai arrived and announced briskly: "I am teaching at Jawaharlal Nehru University, New Delhi. I am researching on stem cell scenario in India. I would like to know about your research. If you have time now, I may sit down or if you wish, I may come later."

We have not known this gentleman before. It was rather sudden and with certain surprise that I looked at him. However, we have always respected professors in sure belief that those who commit themselves to a lifetime of study on a particular subject are the professors at universities. A plethora of universities and deemed universities that have appeared across India has vulgarized the spirit of professorship, but not in our minds. We respect professors of whatever brand and from whatever deemed university. However, Jawaharlal Nehru University is a special kind of its own. Spread across several acres of land with multiple gates and several faculties, at this university, professors believe that they teach students; however, students educate the professors and the vice chancellors. And, if you belong to JNU, you must have been a leftist. A student graduated from JNU, working for *Times of India*, gave us a wide coverage thinking that we may have been a card holding leftist.

So we welcomed Prof. Desai pushing aside a couple of scientists from the office. We asked Prof. Desai, "What would you like to know? We are small researchers in private domain. Stem cell is a very wide field. Yet, we aim at finding a product with mesenchymal stem cells."

Prof. Desai asked simple questions. It was clear that he was not an investigating journalist. He had already collected data from several researchers across India and their institutions, including private companies if that was a platform.

It is difficult to guess what about us would have impressed Pranav Desai. One thing was sure about us is that we never hesitate to disclose, in honest, candid, and clear mode, be it Nayantara from Geneva or a journalist from India or Chicago, or be it Pranav Desai. That had led to the discussion about the regulations and further forward to ethics. At conclusion Prof. Desai asked, "Have you studied guidelines published by ICMR for stem cell research?"

"Yes, from 2006 onwards, every time that ICMR revised it."

"If there are several revised editions, would it not imply that there was confusion with the authors?"

"We are ashamed to confess that independent India has not contributed to a single drug discovery. Those Indians who won Nobel Prizes after independence were researching abroad. We would like ICMR to publish a list of researches that they have promoted and a catalogue of research that they have thwarted. Rajni Vyas was funded by ICMR way back in the 1960s. Her research ended with a negative result that pap smear is not a cost effective method of prevention of cervical cancer. However, with respect to ICMR guidelines, we inform them year after year about our on-going research interests. They have yet to grant recognition to our ethics committee for stem cell research. We do not worry."

About a year later, Prof. Desai sent us a copy of his publication. There was no high scholastic erudition: simply narration of what was going on in India at the time. But attached along with was an invitation to deliver a key note address to the conference that JNU was sponsoring along with King's College of London, with counterparts as Prof. Alex Faulkner.

Dr. Rupa Dave came along to the conference. She provided a poignant insight into nuances about regulating stem cell research. She raised a counter point that when the world knowledge pool about stem cell research is so overflowing with beneficial effects of regeneration with stem cell, how unethical would it be to deny its access to patients who need it? I completed the key note address with the proofs that trigerminal translation of mesenchymal stem cells is indeed possible.

Presentation by Prof. Alex Faulkner from King's College of London was a dénouement. He said that in UK and Western Europe there is yet no single stem cell product on the horizon. A couple of companies in France have successfully produced large scale dressings. The biological dressings have homologous keratinocytes—epithelial skin cells. Their use is for a limited time and has to be frequently changed. Large treatment centres for burn patients in USA and a few in UK has found them to be life saving.

We were holding our breath to hear the presentation from ICMR representatives. At the conclusion of the first day, it was announced that ICMR representative has withdrawn participation. No loss it was to be, since her slot was allotted as an additional slot to Dr. Geeta Shroff. We have known Dr. Geeta Shroff as a maverick. She has been treating incurable conditions such as Spinal cord injury, Diabetes, Multiple sclerosis, Parkinson's disease, Cardiac conditions, and Cerebral palsy. We had seen a patient referred from Vadodara with Spinal Injury that returned with a remarkable surprise recovery.

As Geeta Shroff presented, everyone in the audience sat straight with rapt attention. Most of her data was about treatment of spinal cord injuries. She did not have to elaborate on the nature of the injuries to the vertebral column nor did she mention about the type of injury to the spinal cord. Her presentation ran overtime to be taken up further on the next day.

Dr. Geeta Shroff demonstrated that, following treatment with stem cells, spinal cord injury patients were able to walk; some had crutches but a few had no support. We inquired that in an earlier series reported from All India Institute of Medical Sciences, the results were negative. Dr. Geeta stood firm on her ground. "I have only my results to demonstrate and defend." Professors from King's College, namely Prof. Brian Salter and Prof. Alex Faulkner asked her about the type of stem cells and regulatory approvals. Dr. Geeta refused to be drawn in this domain. Nor did she demonstrate the images about other conditions like Parkinson's disease or Cerebral Palsy. But she extended an invitation: Everybody was invited at her clinic at the conclusion of the Conference to see the patients under treatment.

We had undertaken a proof of concept study with spinal cord injury patients. The patients would range from a near contusion to hemi-section of the spinal cord or a complete trans-section. They may have undergone operative surgery to evacuate blood collection and repair fractured vertebrae. The repair in spinal cord is well understood; though complex in nature.

Grossly speaking, there are two types of neurons in the spinal cord. The motor neurons transmit the impulses of the motor cortex to the muscles of the body, while the sensory neurons convey the sensation to the brain. Each neuron is of specific size and its location is also well defined. Soon after disruption, neuronal cell nucleus sends information to the disrupted end to begin repair whereby the central portion of the cell, extending downwards from the nucleus, known as axon starts regeneration with prolongation, but the spontaneous regeneration ends here. At the site of the injury, there will be organization of the hematoma and invasion by numerous fibroblasts. The proliferating axon will most likely be trapped in such a chaos that its reunion to its own ruptured distal end is highly unlikely. Moreover, the disrupted end undergoes degeneration that affects only axon, leaving its sheath intact. This is intricately understood and is known as Wallarian degeneration. However, how would a proliferating axon connect to its empty sheath may be a micro-molecular engineering. That it does happen, even in isolated cases is a proved positive. But, what would the stem cells may be even of embryonic type contribute, by what properties may not be deciphered for a long time. In human beings, it may be an indefinite time and to evolve the understanding of reparative process with stem cells will need numerous scientists experimenting with various species of animals for a long, long duration. While the scientific hunger for the quest of knowledge for the sake of knowledge will be insatiable, would a clinician wanting to help his patients be non-satisfied that the patient is benefited for sure?

The process is intense up to 6 weeks but continues up to about

9 months when it completely ceases. Even in such an instance, we have come across one instance of regeneration that cannot be explained on the basis of existing knowledge. A young patient paralyzed for about 18 months down below the waist approached us with a carload of relatives. We explained them the academics and declined treatment. They refused to leave our premises, pleading that they have accepted that failure is most likely—almost certain.

There were decubitous ulcers—pressure sores on the buttocks as well as on one foot, on the heel where bone was exposed. We cleaned up the septic areas. Umbilical cord derived mesenchymal stem cells were injected on the edges of the ulcers as well as poured with drops on the base of the ulcers. Soon there was healthy granulation tissue. This was grafted with pinch graft. Pinch grafts also would have carried some stem cells that are contained at the basal layer of the dermis.

There was complete acceptance of the grafts. Pressure sores healed. Thereafter, the patient was treated with autologous bone marrow derived mesenchymal stem cells and umbilical cord derived stem cells intrathically. Umbilical cord blood derived mononuclear stem cells along with very small embryonic like stem cells from umbilical cord blood were injected intravenously.

The patient regained control over micturition and defecation. His sensations recovered at a rapid pace, so rapid as not to be explainable as per the known standards of sensory recovery. Sensory recovery progresses not more than 1 millimeter per day.

The patient was resituated with occupational therapies so as to man a counter at his home shop.

A relative of the patient from the United States donated a handsome amount to stem cell research.

It seemed that Dr. Geeta had hijacked all the interest from the conference. The afternoon sessions drew scant attendance and presentations from the representatives of Drug Controller General of India and some professors of pharmacology were lackluster.

We asked Dr. Geeta to show the type of stem cells that she had used. Her reply was that her scientists had left and the laboratory was closed. But surely there was wonder and amazement to see some of the patients undergoing physiotherapy who have been paralyzed before treatment. Though we would have liked to see other types of patients undergoing neuro-restoration, this was no less a reward. A professor from Jawaharlal Nehru University concluded: "Dr. Geeta, if I were to question you, we will need another conference about the academic processes and implicated ethics etc. but if I were to have a spinal cord injury, I would ask the ambulance to carry me to your clinic for sure and I will leave the treatment in your hands with whatever kind of stem cell that you might be utilizing."

Dr. Geeta did not comment further. Our emails remain unanswered. We came to know that in March 2020, 3 companies manufacturing equipments for stem cell isolation and culture sponsored a semi-academic felicitation for women researchers doing stem cell therapy. Dr. Geeta's presentation was based on same clinical material. Shall we conclude that let there be several violations of regulatory guidelines, even if one patient like ours or a researcher like Dr. Geeta produces beneficial results, let the Pundits ponder, as long as no harm is done!

15
Even Pay to Publish, Since It is Addiction

I gave up the academic teaching job at Medical College, Baroda in 1969. Rajni followed in 1973. Her mode of resignation from the academic job is also a paramount proof of our total identity as one. The reporting time at the clinical wards in Sir Sayaji Hospital, Vadodara was at 8:30 A.M. When both of us were working at the medical college, even when I was the head of the unit, I would push off by 8:20 from home; invariably Rajni will be left alone to wind up the breakfast table. If Rupa would not have gone to kindergarten school, she will have to face a few difficult emotional moments before she can be handed over to the babysitter. This would mean that Rajni will invariably be late. The learned professor and the head of the department were at their best as the gatekeepers. He would note the arrival time for every staff member. Rajni would be told day after day: You are once again late today and the two of them will walk to the wards while he will continue the bickering further.

Rajni had worked with tough taskmasters at work. She had endured working conditions of more than 100 hours a week. This bickering also she can easily shrug off. But when we sit down for lunch, everyday she will recount the same sad story of the professors bickering.

Rajni had brought this matter to the attention of her chief, university professor, Dr. Thakorbhai Patel. Instead of help, he was indignant. "You full-timers behave like *Pantojis*. Why do you not rise to the level of your proven status? You will be one of the first few

Ph.D. holders in India in your subject. Your research on the blood volume studies in third trimester of pregnancy in anaemic women with less than 4 grams is unique. No parallel in world literature. Why don't you brush aside the meaningless remarks by the professors?"

Rajni had understood that she should live with the situation. She has immense patience and tolerance. But there can always be a last straw that will break the camel's back.

Once, she had very heavy emergency week. The hospital drained the patients from several districts all around Vadodara. The obstetric delivery patients very routinely brought to Sir Sayaji General Hospital; at times with rupture of uterus. Such emergency operations, at times over-highly anaemic patients were life saving situation. Rajni had hardly slept a few hours for 7 continuous nights. On the following day, when Rajni narrated the same story, I saw her wet eyes.

And I decided this is no more. I knew that Rajni would not agree. Over the last few years, we have published more than 50 research papers. While I had detoured, Rajni had a precious aim to be a professor. That she had achieved, but the location was to be at Jamnagar. Now she had more than the requisite experience and post of the professor at Medical College, Vadodara was advertised.

However, my mind was made up. That afternoon only, I personally handed over a resignation letter, with a fake signature, signed as 'Rajni Vyas' in the office.

Next morning, Rajni had a pleasant surprise. She was late as usual. The high professors looked at her and looked down. She wondered, no more reminders! Professor conducted her to the office. He asked, "Rajni, why is this?" and showed the letter.

Rajni wondered, is he going to give me a warning in writing this time? She took the letter and could not stop from uttering, "Oh no!"

Professor asked, "So you said oh no. Do you want to withdraw it?"

By this time, Rajni had gathered up the situation. She said, "No, my mind is made up. I want to quit. I don't want to give reasons, please oblige me by forwarding it with favourable remarks."

From that morning after, there was peace for Rajni for about 6 months. The higher authorities accepted her resignation; but to be relieved only after 6 months! Strange are the ways of government functioning and so are the ways of destiny deciding the destination with time specification! At home, Rajni ventilated her aggrievement. Well, the dice is already thrown. Let the barking dogs bark now, if they so choose. She would now have to quit the pristine pure innocence of academic life and will have to jump into turbulent waters of private practice. No regrets: she will measure up to it. She was sorry only on one count; she has been relentlessly persistent in publishing the research. She said, "We have acquired an addiction for research and publishing. How shall we cope with this situation?"

I replied, "We shall derive satiety for this addiction with periodic publication; maybe till such a time that we exist. Let there be no push and drive to publish for promotion. Let this addiction be *Saraswati Puja*."

We have tried to live up to this resolve: Rajni with more spectacular success than mine. What would have been her Ph.D. thesis got published in the British Journal. Her seminal contribution on unexplained reproductive failure was refused by American Journal. Later with eloquent plagiarism, it was published by the Australian editor in Australian Journal.

When we sent three articles, in a series, on unexplained reproductive failure, the editor had asked Rajni, "How old are you?"

Thus research and publication, apart from being an addiction, has become a magnificent obsession with us.

Therefore, when we received an invitation to contribute for publication, it was a big delight. It was like offering free heroin to an opium addict. We reproduced a very enticing letter from a Chinese editor, now publishing from USA and UK both, as follows. The name of the journal has been changed.

"Dear Dr. Bhaskar Vyas,

I came across your paper "Reversal of Hair Greying following Autologous Adipose Mesenchymal Stem Cell Transplantations. A Coincidental Finding" and felt that your work is distinctive for this research domain. This research may indeed prove to be significant to fellow researchers and scientists working in the same discipline.

Taking note of your research interests which matches with our journal domain, may I know more about your current research work? Like we can also develop a network of eminent researchers of your stream worldwide.

As your research work comes under the scope of our journals, I cordially invite you to send your future research articles/papers for publication to Global Journal of Science Frontier Research, DOI: 10.17406/GJSFR.

Regards,
Editor,
Department of Natural Science"

The letter ended with a brief introduction to the Journal. We were excited. But, Anant Marathe had a contrary opinion. He said, "This kind of so-called international or global journals are journals in search of researchers. An open-access journal on the internet costs so much lesser to publish than a hard-copy. We will be lured with various promises. Once we are in the trap, see what happens."

But I argued, "They are promising to publish without payment."

Rajni and I worked overtime for a week and chiselled out an article. Anant Marathe was happy. He said, "Do send it over."

We received prompt acknowledgement. But surprises were to follow. The surprise was in form of a demand asking for payment after acceptance of the article. Yes, we had misunderstood. There was no charge for formatting and typesetting. But, the rest of the charges do apply!

"Dear Dr. Vyas,

We thank you very much for sending your original research article/research paper/review paper and entrusting us to launch it worldwide. In connection with this, please note that every submitted paper will be examined by two peer reviewers to grade it for publication.

In this regard, please note that every submitted paper is double-blind reviewed by peer reviewers and board members. Acceptance, update suggestion, or rejection depends on their comments. The author is requested to pay only after receiving an acceptance letter for the paper. If any improvement is suggested, the author is asked to upgrade and resubmit the paper. The entire process is expected to be completed within a month. We will try to send you a live tracking link three or four working days. You can use that link to track and update your paper without logging in.

We shall be glad to assist you in case you need any clarification.

With warm regards,

Manuscript Executive
Manuscript Department."

"Dear Dr. Vyas,

The Article Processing Charges are USD 938 for "Global Journal of Science Frontier Research." This includes all the charges like fees for two Peer Reviewers (USD 469 × 2 reviewers = USD 938), the cost of Hard Copy of Journal (USD 50), Postal Charges, etc.

Since you belong to Research Promoting Zone, Special Article Processing Charges considered for you are USD 106, instead of USD 938. So you can pay in INR/PKR/BDT etc. (Discounted charges for Zambia, Central African Republic, Afghanistan, Maldives, India, Pakistan, Nepal, Bangladesh, Sri Lanka, & Bhutan).

The author is requested to pay only after receiving an Acceptance Letter of the paper."

In 1992, we published our first book towards holistic health. This was with self-finance. While I was in UK, I approached some commercial publishers. One responder had said that even Bernard Shaw, in his early career was published by them. Howsoever, high it may have been, we have been averse to vanity publication. Therefore, regardless of the merit, we would not like to pay this internationally acclaimed journal to publish our article. We felt cheated, but they clarified, formatting and typesetting were offered free. That did not include publication and fees for their reviewers! How clever ! It was as good as free entry, only exit charge.

We were not expecting any payments to be made. So we replied,

"Dear Dr. Lenzi, Dr. Wu

Thank you for acknowledging the receipt for our submitted article. We would like to clarify as follows:

We have understood that we are invited. Thereby we are not agreeable to pay any amount whatsoever.

With regards,

Bhaskar Vyas,
Chairman,
Total Potential Cells Pvt. Ltd.,
Vadodara, India."

They replied,

"Dear Dr.,
This is to bring in your kind information:

(1) In the light of our "Human Resource Development Division" view, it is very hard for us to provide any discount on your paper.

(2) Being an "Open Access Journal", we provide completely free access to the journals. Hence, the circulation and readers of our Journal are highest which reflects that it is most widely read and of course, this is the best and most preferred way to communicate research work with the world. As every process and function requires funds to meet the expenditures. The profit-making organizations ask the readers to pay to read the journals. However, such a method reduces the number of readers significantly and is widely known as close cabin publication, while "Open Access Journals" provide free access to the complete paper, but are compelled to ask their Authors to pay fees to meet the expenditures.

Open Access should be seen as a means of accelerating scientific discovery by providing free and unrestricted access to scientific knowledge *via* the Internet. An essential role of Open Access is the long-term preservation of peer-reviewed scholarly journal articles and research data. Open Access is not only used for journal articles but is also being implemented to theses, scholarly monographs, and book chapters. Promotion of Open Access is very crucial to encourage innovation, socio-economic development, and the flow of knowledge around the world. As such, Open Access can be defined as an instrument ultimately used for public welfare to stimulate the growth of global science, as well as maintain the quality of scientific achievements at the same time.

Restricted access to research findings and scientific discovery through subscription and pay-per-view journals will only impede communication through the scientific community. Also, limited access can also hamper the education and dissemination of scientific knowledge to the aspiring younger generations who are keen to pursue a career in science. Increased productivity and development of science can only be achieved by diffusing knowledge and providing the facilities for creating permanent repositories such as Open Access.

Please feel free to contact us in case of any queries.

With Warm Regards,
Jennifer Fishburn
Account Manager
Billing Department"

Our reply was,

"Dear sirs,

Thanks. We understand now. We appreciate your situation.

Our situation is that we are unable to pay any amount.

We received some comment from the reviewers. We are willing to accept and will send revised article if and when you think you will publish it without any payment from our side.

With regards,

Bhaskar Vyas,
Corresponding author."

Even bartering is international now and no shame to barter for literary products. The journal business manager scaled down the demand as follows:

"Dear Dr. Vyas,

Sorry Sir, best we can do is 2212 INR without hardcopy.

In this case, should we proceed for withdrawal?"

Rajni and I discussed to differ. I would have liked not to pay as a matter of principle. Rajni's view was that we have ourselves gained further insights. There reviewers have taken immense pains to write elaborately. They have given our research 'A' grade.

The amount to pay was not much and the principal to be compromised was no more so sanctimonious. So we agreed.

"Dear Friends and the team,

Thanks.

We shall remit the amount 2212 INR online to your ICICI bank account.

Regards,

Bhaskar Vyas,

Corresponding author."

Both the reviewers have conducted dissecting division into 7 main categories. They are further divided into several sub-divisions.

Theme, Extensibility of Research, Application of Research, Structural and Compilation Gradation of Article, Interactivity, Title, Abstract and Keywords, Introduction Section, Material & Methods Section, Article Content, Results Section, Discussion/Conclusion Section and Total & Grade. This further extended to (we wondered, good heavens, how much time would they have had to spend even if they were to enter on a template!) Integrity & Analysis of Theme, Depth of the Research, Logical Conclusions, Relevance of the Article, Flexibility of input data etc.

We shared the experience with Dr. Umakant Dave. In his inimitable mindfulness mode, he had understood both the sides of the situation. He said, "These kinds of open access journals are useful to the beginners. They help them by publishing when an access to the professional discipline journal would be hard for them. They help to build their curriculum vitae. That you do not need. But, they have provided some satiety by providing a small dose of 'heroin' for your magnificent obsession!"

16
Eureka! A New Drug Discovery on the Horizon!

Nobel Prize is customarily awarded to basic sciences. Even mathematics and economics are excluded though awarded through a different route. Drug discoveries are rarely awarded.

Advances in chemistry are basic to drug discovery, since modern medicine heavily relies on discovering newer molecules to serve as therapeutic agents. Discovery of the structure of benzene ring by Kekule happened with a story. There is an ancient Greek symbol 'ouroboros' that depicts a snake holding its own tail with its mouth. Kekule had a dream where he expanded this symbol to 6 snakes and conceptualized a hectagonal structure with carbon atom as a bond. We now know this as the structure of benzene and it has gone on to provide a basic structure for organic chemistry. New molecules begun to be synthesized so as to effectively treat various kinds of diseases. Therefrom most of the newer chemical molecules including for therapeutic use are derived from.

Let us browse through some significant molecules which are the main ingredients of ground breaking medications.

Aspirin (chemical ingredient—acetylsalicylic acid) began to be used from the middle of the nineteenth century. It began to be used widely as a pain killer and anti inflammatory drug. If chloroquine had been available in the first half of the twentieth century, it is possible that Napoleon may not have lost the war against Russia! The pinnacle of achievement of synthesizing a molecule is exemplified by synthetic insulin molecule that is now being used as a drug. The drug is composed of numerous amino acids that are chained together to prepare a protein molecule—insulin. Banting (a Canadian orthopaedic surgeon) is credited with success in isolating the active substance from the pancreas. Crucially it is generally accepted that insulin has not been used in animals before being used in human patients.

One of the first drugs used to combat bacterial infections for sulfocetamide.

Diseases such as gonorrhea and syphilis are near extinction, primarily because of penicillin.

Alexander Fleming, a professor of microbiology at St. Marys Hospital, London accidentally discovered penicillin. He was culturing microbes in petri dishes and left for two weeks while he was on vacation. When he returned, he happened to discover that there were no microbes around a mold on one of the petri dishes. It was as if the mould had secreted something to inhibit the growth of the colony. On further investigation, it turned out to be what we know now as a strain of penicillin.

In his own words, "One sometimes finds what one is not looking for. When I woke up just after dawn, I certainly did not plan to revolutionize all medicine by discovering the world's first antibiotic, or bacteria killer. But I guess that was exactly what I did." This revolutionized the practice of medicine. Antibiotics have played a major role in helping doctors combat microbial infections. Since the discovery of penicillin, successively stronger antibiotics have been engineered and made available. Unfortunately, now the real challenge is that they rapidly lose their effectiveness because of development of resistant strains of micro-organisms.

India has a rich heritage of Ayurvedic medicine. It is unfortunate that its contribution and knowledge has not been investigated in the same manner as modern medicine. Sporadic interest has shown how extensive the knowledge of this ancient system is... In 1950s, a plant that has been used since ancient times to lower the blood pressure was subjected to scrutiny and study. Rauwolfia, described in *Charak Samhita* as *Sarpagandha* was used widely in the Ayurvedic system for a variety of uses, most commonly as a tranquiliser. After analysis, a new drug, Recerpine was made from the derivative of

Rauwolfia to be used as an antihypertensive agent; but was soon replaced with more effective chemically derived molecules.

Another chemotherapeutic drug; Vincristine is derived from a common garden plant, Vinca Rosea or Periwinkle. This is patented now by China; although the plant is there in almost every home in the kitchen garden in India! It is a common plant that grows easily in India amongst other sub-tropical countries. When vincristine was isolated from this plant, lily (the original pharmaceutical company who manufactured it) held a monopoly on its manufacture.

Biodiversity in the vegetable kingdom in India is immense. There is huge potential for repertoire for researchers to follow modern scientific models of drug discovery through this vegetable kingdom.

Most human beings are likely to need some kind of drugs during their life-span. Every year the population on the Earth is increasing. That contributes to the expansion of the market size. Thus, pharma-industry as of today is only second to that of the defence equipments.

It was not always so. There was a pharma-company that was benevolent to human beings. The founders of the company had a vision that it will be innovations and research that will propel the progress of business. Burroughs Wellcome Pharmaceutical Company is no more in existence but the Wellcome Trust is now helping scientists early in their careers develop as independent investigators and to advance in basic biomedical sciences. Fortunately for mankind, both the founders of the company Sir Henry Wellcome and Silas Burroughs did not have children. When Glaxo bought over Burroughs Wellcome, most of the funds went to Burroughs Wellcome Fund, which is one of the largest charity foundations. This was a unique model and it is extremely unlikely to be repeated in the current climate that we live in.

In India as in the rest of the world, pharmaceutical companies have grown exponentially in size as well as financially. They are content to simply fulfil their obligations by being compliant to socially responsible funding. In the present century, all *isms* have become *wasms.* It goes without saying that business is for profit and without apologies to the yesteryears, profit has seized to be a dirty word in India as well. Whatever may be the curses inflicted on various kinds of *isms,* the saving grace for capitalism is benevolence. Political philosophy including discussions and debates on *isms* and *wasms* is a far cry from the story of stem cells. Yet, it does concern the future of stem cell research to the extent that there is well known resistance to this kind of regenerative medicine research since it may affect the status of current in vogue expensive drugs.

With this prelude, at the onset we had known that we were too small to arrive at any drug discovery. We were satisfied with the motto that though large is powerful, *small is beautiful.* And we have derived strength from a quote from the Dalai Lama, "If you think you are too small to make a difference, think of sleeping with only one mosquito around." However, we did not mean to cause disturbance to anyone, for sure.

When Bangladesh became a freshly carved independent nation, population and poverty were abounding. A maverick activist health minister practically banished the multinational pharmaceutical companies from the country. He ruthlessly narrowed the list of 'must needed' medicines to 100. He supported marketing of these drugs with their generic names so as to bring down the prices at bare minimum. This ensured that people could afford the medicines that they needed to regain or maintain health. But, this may be considered a utopian dream as of now.

Every citizen of the world has a fundamental right to freedom, equality and liberty. Most of the people would want to prolong their life span as long as possible. Along with the desire to increase life span, the demand to look good and youthful is insatiable. Therefore, the need for discovery of new drugs, particularly those that can regenerate and rejuvenate is ever-present.

With this scenario, the government has a duty to protect people from hoax claims and fake practices. When we started our careers, medical practice was considered to be both an art and science. Some doctors would even 'smell' a patient or just hold the wrist and count the pulse and will have a hunch as to what was ailing the patient.

Our textbooks of practice of surgery began with an inscription such as, "I dress the wounds of my patients; God heals them." Attraction of white blood corpuscles to the site of infection was attributed by theologists universally as an evidence of Divine Design.

God no more exists in medical textbooks. Current medical practice has emerged to be evidence-based practice of medicine. Plethoras of laboratory investigations are available that most of the times can give a correct evidence based diagnosis. Once established, it leaves little room for practicing artful medicine: the usage of the indicated drug with well established dosage modules works out like a mathematical equation. This is the pinnacle of achievement by modern medicine. The honing of stem cells at the site of need is understood as engineered by the properties of molecules present and by the properties of cytokines—biochemical substances secreted by stem cells.

The process of discovering a new drug begins with a concept based on empirical evidence generated out of basic scientific research. The concept is then subjected to animal experiments. When the animals do not have a diseased condition, such as, say fibrocystic disease of the lung, a research model that can replicate fibrocystic disease of the lung in animals is reproduced. The animal species may range from a little mouse to large animals, may be even a deer (remember, one and only clone model devised was Dolly the sheep?). With successful results verified against controlled placebo (placebo is an innocuous inert substance having no physiological properties) trials are conducted. Thereafter, independent ethics committee approvals are needed. Ethics committees have to be approved by government agencies exercising authority to regulate drug control. In India, Central Drug Standard Control Organization and Drug Controller General of India are authorized for approval. In addition, Indian Council of Medical Research issues periodical guidelines for stem cells research. This step as has been our experience is where there is a major road block. Let us explain:

We have approached these agencies several times in the course of our work. We would not like to go into great detail; suffice it to say that the narration will surely attract praise for the patience, tolerance and persistence and evoke great sadness at the sordid face of Mother India. We have constantly worked with the slogan that not failure, but low aim is a crime. Some may say, 'How sad!' If it was only to express sadness, even failure, we would surely have tried. We have several times mused on Shelly, "*Our sweetest songs are those that tell of saddest thought*" or we have sung along with Rabindranath Tagore, the songs of the defeated.

We trust that the sadness and the sordidness eventually will disappear. And so, let us pass it on without further discussion. At the bottom line, a certain fact does emerge that there must have been a solid reason as to why independent India, independent with more than 70 years has not been successful in discovering a new drug.

Our surmise to find an answer to such a question is simple. Indian system of medicine was based on profundity of wisdom of Charak…. On the contrary, present day medical practice is now under the heavy burden of Helsinki Declaration.

We briefly state some guidelines of the Helsinki Declaration. A global association of medical doctors, World Medical Association has promulgated guidelines for conducting a clinical trial on humans: The importance of the objective must outweigh the risks and burdens to the research subjects. This is elementary and would surely be followed without additional burden by an Indian researcher whose basic archetype is to fear God. The protocol for clinical trials should also include information regarding funding, sponsors, institutional affiliations, potential conflicts of interest, incentives for subjects and information regarding provisions for treating and/or compensating subjects who are harmed as a consequence of participation in the research study. This is also easily achieved by Indian researchers.

What is really formidable for India is multi-staging of the clinical trials. A new drug discovery involves formulating a preamble to the concept. This will be based on global research survey of what has already been established with animal experimentation. Proof of concept may further need to be buttressed with proof of concept studies in one or more species of animals and at least 6 human subjects. Further regulatory clearances from the ethics committee as well as drug control authorities have to be taken.

A statistical validation for the results can only be explained when the number of patients subjected to stage 1 of the clinical trial is more than 20. Another parameter may have to be included for statistical validity. That is randomized double blind controlled clinical trial that may use placebos or a less effective tool already in use as a blind control. Clinical trial stage 2, 3 and 4 extend from 50-500 patients. Further evidence needs to be generated with a multi-centric trial.

The patient must not have to carry any financial burden. Risk-burden, in case of any adverse event, must be compensated financially to the patients.

Stem cell research is regulated in India by Indian Council of Medical Research. From 2006 to 2017, they have published several editions of the guideline. The guidelines do not have any legal authority. We have endeavoured several times, year after year to register a clinical trial with the drug control authorities (DCGI) in India and have succeeded only once.

To our pleasant surprise, we found that we could register our proposed clinical trials online with Drug Controller General of India. We constituted an institutional ethics committee and with their approval, we have uploaded more than a dozen clinical trials on DCGI website. I must confess that patience is not one of my virtues! Hence pending approval we began one of the clinical trials. Imagine our amusement when we got retrospective approval for this trial, 3 years after the original application !

One of our trials included working with stem cells derived from fatty tissue. Several insights on the horizon have appeared from the isolation, culture and expansion of these stem cells.

We are able to process about 1000cc lipoaspirate, within a few hours to have a few ccs of stromal vascular factor. It contains a combination of mesenchymal stem cells, a few hemopoietic stem cells and other cells such as endothelial precursor cells, macrophages, smooth muscle cells, lymphocytes, pericytes, and pre-adipocytes. While we contemplated that this minimally manipulated product may as well be utilized since it contains large number of (approximately 30-35 per cent Mesenchymal Stem cells) facilitation happened from CDSCO: Stromal Vascular Factor was proclaimed as a drug in 2017. When this was put for comments in public domain, ICMR asserted that stem cells and their derivatives fall under definition of 'Drug' as per the Drugs and Cosmetics Act, 1945, and are further categorized as 'Investigational New Drug (IND)' or 'Investigational New Entity (INE)' when used for clinical application. A similar statement was also issued in a letter to DCGI from International Society for Stem Cell Research.... The letter stated, "The ISSCR represents more than 4,000 stem cell researchers around the world, including many in India. We are pleased to see that CDSCO is joining other global regulators in endeavouring to develop strong rules to improve the regulation of new stem cell therapies and help assure patients these products are safe and effective. We urge CDSCO to consider the revisions, which will further protect patients from unproven products and procedures falsely marketed as stem cell therapies." Obviously, their bias was in favour of *strong rules*. Discovery of a new drug from Indian research does not seem to be likely in the foreseeable future in the face of formidable rules and regulations. As estimated by Pfizer, new drug discovery in 2020 would cost around $130 million.

A moth in utter wilderness, may dream to be a star! That shall never happen. But, a moth may metamorphosize to be a butterfly. This remained our aspiration.

When we got funded for translating adipose derived MSCs to insulin producing cells, naïve as we were, we put our research on the clinical trial domain webpage. We like the fact that computer applications behave like idiot savants. Whatever might be the understanding of semantics by computer, or let us say, by some administrative mischance, our clinical trial to conduct a proof of concept study got approved! I suffered from peripheral neuritis due to diabetes. I felt as if a million small ants were marching up and down my limbs. All known treatments for neuritis did not bring me any relief.

Rajni, (I say it again and again,) is an epitome of patience, perseverance, persistence and forbearance. In contradiction, my personality is prone to proactive action with emotional inputs. True to my impulsive self, I decided that I would be the first and perhaps only patient for a trial to treat this condition with ADMSC.

I was fearless of any adverse reactions since my symptoms were intolerable. I deemed myself to be the researcher, investigator and the patient. I requested Rajni and the rest of my family members to assist and assess my treatment and its response. I am proud to join the privileged group of very few researchers who have tried their research on themselves.

So severe was my discomfort that I refused to listen to the protests of my family. I proceeded to write up the protocol that we would use for the treatment. *Aha*! It is more than 5 years since; I have not experienced even a single kind of electrocutting spark like jerks anywhere in my body. This is a success story for the stem cells.

Whilst I have benefited by this procedure, it did put my immediate and extended family through an emotional rollercoaster. Rajni and Nirupa (our younger daughter) were unwavering in their support but kept their fears to themselves.

Rupa our elder daughter insisted that she remain present.

Dr. Chitralekha Dave arrived from Surat for implementing the administration of stem cells and to provide moral support. In the morning, I was at a corporate hospital for lipoaspiration which was done under local anaesthesia. As soon as the procedure was over, I insisted on discharge from the hospital with the pretext that, "Hospitals are dirty with invisible microbes that may include methicillin resistant staphylococci bacteria and others such as esterechia coli, H. pertusis and others. Home is surely a better place." I threatened to walk out against medical advice at which point my family and the staff at the hospital reluctantly agreed to take me home. The stem cells were administered at home.

On the next day, I was comfortable with minimal side effects from the drugs. The family was watching a show on television at about 9 P.M. I told Rupa that "I am having a feeling of slight pain on the left side of the chest."

Rupa is working in Britain where the ethos is to take abundant precaution. Acting sharply, in a few minutes she set several wheels in motion. Before I could protest about going back into hospital, my grandsons helped me down four flights of stairs and Nirupa drove me to the hospital. Dr. Dilip Trivedi, Rajni's brother, (senior eminent surgeon in Mumbai) was able to board the overnight train to Baroda and arrived the next morning. I had to spend the night in intensive care unit. Where was the pain? It had disappeared before I sat in the car ! Several investigations and constant monitoring of vital parameters revealed total normalcy. All the same, I had to spend one more day in the hospital for abundant precaution.

Dilip was furious. For the first time he reprimanded me. I remained silent, being at the receiving end. Dilip shot out several volleys of academic questions. "Do you know that there is also a phenomenon called 'host *vs.* graft' reaction? If this were to happen even now subsequently, how shall we take care of you?" When he came to know that I had planned a second session with cultured and expanded mesenchymal stem cells, he ordered them to be thrown away.

Maybe the second shot would have helped me even more. Autologous stem cells will certainly not cause a 'host *vs.* graft' reaction. But there was no arguing the fact that with my brashness, I had roughed up the kind feeling of family members. To date, they have always tolerated this with forbearance, but this time I was left with no illusions that I would have to answer God Almighty if I acted with brazen bashfulness again."

This solitary personal verification is enough of evidence for us. I can understand that the reader may not agree with the proposed method or doubt that one case is of validation for treatment. If we ever have the means to do so, I would aspire to conduct a clinical trial for this indication.

Multiple collateral benefits happen to accrue from really diminutive number of diabetic patients who have been part of our trial workload. A patient having diabetic retinopathy spontaneously reported improvement of the vision in both the eyes. Another showed lowering of blood creatinine levels after stem cell treatment. A juvenile diabetic girl having frequent ketoacidosis attacks had no more ketone bodies in the urine. Yet another juvenile diabetic is now a mother with excellent control of her diabetes 10 years after the first treatment.

What amazes us about the collateral benefits is an incidental finding of grey hair turning black. This happened to me and persists with increased number of black hair even after 5 years. We were casual about reporting this research. Surprisingly, it generated worldwide interest and continues to do so even now in 2020! We received an email from the editor of an international journal, which is mentioned in another chapter. It is published in June 2020 issue. This time, using bioinformatics as a tool, we described in this publication as to how we could bypass so many steps, the scientific methods are omitted but even for a lay reader, the logical elegance will be of interest.

Genesis of this report is due to several requests, initially generated by publication in a regional news magazine, *Gujarat Medical Journal*. We noted, as an accidental finding in our ongoing research on neuro-degenerative diseases treated with Bone Marrow derived Mesenchymal Stem Cells (BM-MSCs) or with Adipose Derived Mesenchymal Stem Cells (ADMSCs). We decided to academically progress the research by publishing it in a journal devoted to stem cell research. This publication in turn has generated global interest and we are receiving reprint requests and the protocols. Meanwhile we have successfully translated ADMSCs to all three germinal layers. Potential is thus expanded to a new drug discovery.

Advances in bioinformatics have so progressed that using computers as a dry laboratory, enormous data can be accessed. We, therefore, report on the progression of our research on MSCs as well as results obtainable with bioinformatics on several cytokines that may have impinged our research.

This accidental finding seems to be pointing towards simultaneous stimulatory effect on a small organ such as a hair follicle. Hair follicles are derived from ectoderm. The hair pigment, melanin will be secreted by glandular cells, which have an endodermic origin! As of now we are unable to explain how black hair growth is seen.

Thus, the research highlights that howsoever ambiguous a finding in research, it should not be given a pass. Nature may appear to be playing dice but it does not.

Had Alexander Fleming given a pass to a chance nonoccurrence of microbial growth in a particular Petri dish, penicillin may not have been discovered. Therefore, every occurrence, howsoever trivial, must be explained. Researchers usually publish positive results. We should derive inference as to how 10 of the 14 patients did not show the positive signs.

This accidental finding has charted a pathway to possible new drug discoveries. The process will take long to go through various stages of clinical trials. Yet, it is established, with additional evidence as presented in this research that it is plausible that ADMSCs may be a futuristic drug.

The research also highlights how bioinformatics shortens the processes that would have taken a long time to establish in a wet laboratory.

Another possibility for the discovery of a new drug from stem cell is based on the property of stem cells to undergo translation to the third germinal layer, which is chondrogeneic translation. Cartilage in the knee joint in old people gets eroded due to multiple factors. When advanced, it is not treatable with any drugs and requires replacement of knee joints. Here also, a mischance happened when we were given permission by the Department of Biotechnology to do clinical trial with 25 patients. We selected 25 such patients who had both the knees affected and could carry out the trial on 50 knees. This was accepted by funding agencies as not any misadventure but a little cleverness for better utilization of funds. We have said this before that this research has provided hope for survival for our future efforts. Such hope will sustain small researchers like us.

However, nature has so ordained that now in 2020, there is an urgent need to find a new drug for Corona virus affected patients. In urgent needs a phrase has emerged, 'compassionate approval'. When this is in context with beneficial effects of stem cells, what better boost can stem cell research have? This we will discuss in the subsequent chapter.

17
If Wishes were Horses, Everybody will Want to Ride: Dream We Must

One can encounter stories regarding wishful thinking all over the globe, across all the cultures. It will be an unfortunate child who has not been told the stories regarding flying horses and charming princesses ! Some of the bestselling books, even in this computer age are those that talk about weird, unbelievable and yet realistic like stories. The sweetest songs have been sung about the dreams lost, yet:

> If wishes were horses, everybody would want to ride,
> Yet, dream we must since dreams do realize!

Researchers across the globe, working in prestigious laboratories, have produced voluminous data concerning the regenerative and rejuvenative properties of several kinds of stem cells. How do the stem cells bring about this change is also rigorously pursued and debated. Some believe that the stem cells may indeed translate to the required kind of cell at that particular site by honing (as the Siberian birds do) to the site where they are required. There is also enough evidence that they produce secretions by themselves—cytokines—that are needed for regeneration at the site or possibly all over the body. This would have been enough to justify their clinical use at the beginning of twentieth century.

Let us explain why feel that this may have been the case !

Acetylsalicylic acid is now an across the counter drug sold as Aspirin or Disprin.

We met Nobel Laureate Martin Evans soon after he was knighted at Cardiff University, Wales in 2008. He was radiating benevolence and modesty so typical of a suave gentleman. He was bemused as to why we would want to meet him?

We said, "We are researchers in stem cells in a very small way from India."

"What are your areas of research?"

"We are looking to find clinical applications of mesenchymal stem cells."

His face lit up further. "This is all that will matter at the end. I was the first to culture mice embryonic stem cells and cultivate them in a laboratory in 1981. I produced an animal model to replicate fibrocystic lung disease.

Of course, that will facilitate further researchers to replicate fibrocystic lung disease and try various drugs and maybe stem cells to arrive at a proof of concept. By this time several animals would have been sacrificed. Of course, Society for Prevention of Cruelty to Animals with their vigilant watch will limit the number of sacrificed animals.

But this is a process that is put in practice so as to safeguard human being before clinical application."

He further continued "As a medical doctor, you would have used aspirin numerous times. Was such a process, beginning today with proof of concept going on to verification of animal models, which then has to be taken to three stages of clinical trials and takes a few years, practiced by Bayer, the pharmaceutical company? Who pioneered its sales in early nineteenth century?

We do not know. But we do know that apart from effectively helping patients with headache, it has several other clinical applications.

You would have known that there are side effects to acetylsalicylic acid such as brain hemorrhage, bleeding in GI tract, etc. some patients have lost their lives. Is the drug banned from clinical use now?

No. Acetaminophen/paracetamol and ibuprofen discovered as a replacement to aspirin are known to damage kidneys. They would have undergone the stipulated drug discovery protocol. Despite these side effects, Ibuprofen is used by the medical profession with caution."

He paused for effect.

We took our cue—"Sir Martin—, we do not understand the point that you are driving at. Would you kindly elaborate?"

"Before my research will be put to use for the benefit of mankind, at least 10 years will elapsed. This will be with a view to protect human beings. But if some kinds of stem cell were to help fibrocystic disease of the lung, and several patients would have lost their lives in the period, is it not unfair to these currently suffering patients who would have otherwise benefited?"

"To my mind, drug discovery process is a utopian idea. It's common knowledge that multinationals have their business interests to protect. They would have spent millions in the quest of a new drug discovery. Hence from idea to implementation is a long winded process.

I believe that the regenerative properties of stem cells have been proved enough. A way should be found so that stem cells can be used within clinical settings as soon as possible."

We were inspired and enthused by the logical arguments by Sir Martin.

Freud's book, '*The Interpretation of Dreams*' published in the last year of the nineteenth century is still a favoured pursuit of psychoanalysis. In the book he postulates that dreams arise from deep unconscious mind and find expression as metaphors. William James took it further beyond the unconscious mind and postulated that there is archetypal memory. It is believed by many people across the globe that dreams may herald and may indeed be harbingers of the events to come. We believe that dreams may also be so programmed that they have a formative power to generate material events. Regardless of hypothesis, it is indeed true that *idea is the first reality*.

Therefore, we visualize that,

- Someday there will be a new dawn so as to benefit the largest number of patients with affordable priced stem cell products.

- A mutual consent by the patient/family of the patient and the drug dispenser/medical doctor will be all that might be necessary to use a stem cell product.
- Helsinki declaration may prevail for the affluent nations. There shall be a new ethical code of conducting clinical trials based on ethics, proclaimed in the *Bhagavad Geeta.*

Of course, quacks abound and should be prevented. However, in a free democratic society, people cannot be stopped from having faith in *fakirs*, *sants* and *mahatmas*. And hidden persuasions can be effectively deployed by hiring proficient people. Advertising as a means of mass communication has graduated to a refined profession.

Stem cell research and therapy in India· including our own, came across a stormy threat in 2014. General elections in India were due. Political parties need funding for their election campaigns.... The situation was saved by a courageous, risk-taking and yet duty conscious Drug Controller General of India, Arunkumar B. Ramteke.

Ramteke put a letter in public domain. He wrote that he is under constant pressure from the health secretary and the health minister to put severe restrictions on stem cell research and therapy. As per the requirements, objections to such a notification had to be filed within 45 days.

We immediately objected to any blanket package of restrictions. We do not know how many stem cell researchers would have objected. Crucially the 45 days ended after the results of the general elections were announced and a new government was sworn in. We personally met Arunkumar B. Ramteke, congratulated and thanked him. Initially modest and reticent to discuss more, when prodded he disclosed that at that time he had put in more than 30 years of service. He was due to retire within 2 months. He had foreknowledge that authorities, even higher than the health minister were interested in stopping stem cell research. It was rumored that if the move was not implemented, Ramteke may be suspended and an ordinance may be promulgated. Ramteke concluded: "I am a small man, risen from the ranks with perseverance to my duties. A suspension at very nearly the end of a stellar service record would be very hard for me and my family. However, I did not support the decision as an individual. Before putting the matter in public domain, I asked myself only one question, "Am I doing my duty as required by the service rules?' When my conscience answered me yes, I did not think any more about the consequences." We salute the spirit of Ramteke and dream of a day when India will have many more public servants like Ramteke.

Support for stem cell treatments also came from across the continents, Barack Obama, the then President of USA put forward a fervent appeal. He said researchers doing profound, in-depth research under microscope and experimenting with animals in the laboratory have enormous time; crucially a patient whose life is under threat cannot wait till conclusive evidence is obtained. Barack Obama relaxed several restrictions imposed by his predecessors that prevented the outgoing flux of stem cell researchers. However, the norms for conducting clinical trial are the same as of today—they take so long to complete.

According to the current standards, a new drug has to be tested under numerous protocols including double blind controlled clinical trials before it can be used. Simply stated, while one group of patients is given the drug under testing, the other group of patients with the same conditions is given a placebo. Statistically significant number of patients must improve and the placebo given patients should be significantly less in improvement and in number then the drug can be said to be effective. It is a well known fact that this takes a lot of time and requires a huge financial investment.

The world currently finds itself in the throes of Covid-19 pandemic. There is no cure available. There is no drug that can eliminate the virus. There is no vaccine to protect against the virus. Survivors from the conditions would have managed to do so with their own immune processes. Since, one of the properties of stem cells immune protection and enhancement, an Israeli firm produced a stem cell product derived from the placenta. It was used by the clinicians at Mt. Sinai Hospital in New York. If the normal regulatory approval were required to be obtained, it may have taken several years. However, a new term emerged: compassionate approval. In the anticipation that such an approval would be granted, the stem cells were administered to 12 critically ill Corona patients. 10 of these came off the ventilators and were subsequently discharged.

"What we saw in the very first patient was that within four hours of getting the cells, a lot of her parameters started to get better", said Dr. Karen Osman, who led the team at Mount Sinai.

The doctor said she was encouraged by the results, though she was hesitant to link the stem cell procedure to her patients' recovery.

"We don't know" if the 10 people removed from ventilators would not have gotten well had they not been given the infusion of the stem cells, she said. "And we would never dare to claim that it was related to the cells."

She explained that a "randomized controlled trial" would be the only way "to make a true comparison".

It is obvious that there can be no repeat run for the cured and discharged patients: the patients would be thankful that they are alive; relatives may have spent or donated some amount that cannot be equated with a life saved. But, the treating doctor has acted with wisdom. Being able to wean and discharge 10 out of 12 patients should amount to a stupendous success story; certainly anybody could be proud of. But, Dr. Karen's response was subdued. Discretion is better than valour. Had Dr. Karen claimed to be responsible for this first time success story about usage of stem cells and favourable results, she would have been subjected to a lot of criticism from her peers and other researchers. By admitting that there has not been a randomized controlled clinical trial to test the efficacy of the stem cells, she ensured that the report would survive the anticipated disapproval. She was satisfied to put on record what actually happened and admitted in advance the limitations.

With such an occurrence, we asked: how far long the ethical yardstick—or the ethical regulatory sword may be wielded? If a double controlled clinical trial would have been given to another 12 patients and if most of them would have died, who should be held responsible?

Therefore, we dream of a day when even an anticipatory compassionate approval may not be needed in a situation where it is plausible that some benefits are likely to ensue from stem cell therapy.

Under the pretext of protecting the people, large scale dictatorships have emerged. This has happened in spite of democratic checks and counter-checks. A government that governs the least is a utopian idea and would surely be the best government. We continue to dream of a day when India wakes up to our dream that stem cell research and therapy will be governed the least in India.

We rewrite the poem by Rabindranath Tagore as follows:

Where the mind is without fear and the head is held high;
No stem cell researcher will ever fear
Persecution, imprisonment or revocation of licence.
Where knowledge and research sharing is done without reserve;
Where the world is united in pursuit of research
Affordable to all in regenerative domain
Where the publications come out from the depth of true research;
Where tireless striving produces reproducible results
Stretching its extension to multiple situations;
Where the clear stream of reason has not lost its way
Into a stereotype aping of the Western models,
In copy and paste prototype
Where the mind is led forward by Nature and God that you may be led
Into ever-widening thought and action
Into that heaven of regenerative medicine, my Father, let my country awake.

Index